Rheumatology

A Clinical Handbook

Feedback, errors and omissions

We are always pleased to receive feedback (good and bad) about our books – if you would like to comment on any of our books, please email info@scionpublishing.com.

We've worked really hard with the authors to ensure that everything in the book is correct. However, errors and ambiguities can still slip through in books as complex as this. If you spot anything you think might be wrong, please email us and we will look into it straight away. If an error has occurred, we will correct it for future printings and post a note about it on our website so that other readers of the book are alerted to this.

Thank you for your help.

Rheumatology

A Clinical Handbook

SECOND EDITION

Mohsin Azam
GP Principal, Torrington Park Group Practice, London

Gabriel Samanta
Medical Student, Imperial College London

Ash Samanta
Emeritus Consultant Rheumatologist, University Hospitals of Leicester

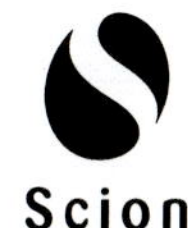

Scion

Second edition published 2025
First edition published 2014

A CIP catalogue record for this book is available from the British Library.

ISBN 9781914961618

Scion Publishing Limited

The Old Hayloft, Vantage Business Park, Bloxham Road, Banbury OX16 9UX, UK
www.scionpublishing.com

Important Note from the Publisher

The information contained within this book was obtained by Scion Publishing Ltd from sources believed by us to be reliable. However, while every effort has been made to ensure its accuracy, no responsibility for loss or injury whatsoever occasioned to any person acting or refraining from action as a result of information contained herein can be accepted by the authors or publishers.

Readers are reminded that medicine is a constantly evolving science and while the authors and publishers have ensured that all dosages, applications and practices are based on current indications, there may be specific practices which differ between communities. You should always follow the guidelines laid down by the manufacturers of specific products and the relevant authorities in the country in which you are practising.

Although every effort has been made to ensure that all owners of copyright material have been acknowledged in this publication, we would be pleased to acknowledge in subsequent reprints or editions any omissions brought to our attention.

Registered names, trademarks, etc. used in this book, even when not marked as such, are not to be considered unprotected by law.

Line artwork by Hilary Strickland Illustration, Bath, UK
Typeset by Medlar Publishing Solutions Pvt Ltd, India
Printed in the UK
Last digit is the print number: 10 9 8 7 6 5 4 3 2 1

Contents

Preface to the second edition ... vii
Preface to the first edition ... viii
Acknowledgments ... ix
Abbreviations ... x

1 Introduction ... 1

2 Specific conditions ... 7
2.1 Rheumatoid arthritis ... 8
2.2 Osteoarthritis ... 15
2.3 Septic arthritis ... 20
Introduction to spondyloarthropathies ... 24
2.4 Psoriatic arthritis ... 25
2.5 Ankylosing spondylitis ... 30
2.6 Reactive arthritis ... 35
2.7 Gout ... 39
2.8 Calcium pyrophosphate disease ... 44
2.9 Vasculitis ... 47
2.10 Giant cell arteritis ... 55
2.11 Polymyalgia rheumatica ... 59
2.12 Systemic lupus erythematosus ... 62
2.13 Polymyositis and dermatomyositis ... 69
2.14 Sjögren's syndrome ... 74
2.15 Scleroderma ... 78
2.16 Fibromyalgia ... 84
2.17 Osteoporosis ... 88
2.18 Paget's disease ... 93

3 Paediatric rheumatology conditions ... 97
3.1 Vitamin D deficiency ... 98
3.2 Juvenile idiopathic arthritis ... 103

4 Investigations ... 109
4.1 Blood tests ... 110
4.2 Immunological tests ... 116

4.3	Synovial fluid analysis	120
4.4	Imaging	123
5	**Pharmacology**	127
5.1	Analgesia	128
5.2	Corticosteroids	133
5.3	Osteoporosis drugs	135
5.4	DMARDs and biological agents	139
6	**OSCEs**	149
6.1	History taking	150
6.2	Examination	153
6.3	Differential diagnosis	158
Appendix	Photograph acknowledgments	161
Index		165

Additional self-assessment questions are available on the Resources tab at:

www.scionpublishing.com/Rheum2.

Preface to the second edition

It is now ten years since the first edition of *Rheumatology – a clinical handbook* was published. Over the years, I have received comments from medical students, newly qualified doctors, trainees in rheumatology and consultant colleagues, who have said how much they enjoyed going through this text. Phrases used have been "a very useful little book", "highly informative", "well set out and sign-posted", "easy to read" and "contains key information". Whilst such encouraging reports are extremely gratifying, at the same time they serve as reminders that the reputation of this book can only be maintained if it is updated, which is what this new edition achieves.

I am very pleased that Mohsin Azam has remained as an author. Mohsin was one of the authors of the original version, at which time he was a medical student in Leicester. He is now a Principal GP in North London. Despite his extremely busy schedule, Mohsin has generously given up much of his time to contribute to developing the new edition, for which I am very grateful.

I am delighted to welcome Gabriel Samanta as a new member to the team of authors. In the interests of openness and transparency I must declare that Gabriel is my son and is a medical student at Imperial College London. Despite his ongoing studies and working on a project as part of his course, he has researched and updated all chapters to provide a first draft which Mohsin and I have carefully reviewed. Gabriel deserves to be commended not only for his hard work but also for his courage and tenacity in working under the watchful (and nagging) influence of his dad!

Earlier readers of *Rheumatology – a clinical handbook* will observe that the format is as before. This is because of the positive feedback received in the past, wherein much credit was placed upon the layout of the chapters and on the colour coding, headings and signposting, all of which were regarded as particularly useful. All chapters have been reviewed and revised as required. The principal changes are updating in respect of new substantive material, immunological investigations, relevant blood tests, imaging, and new treatments that include biologics as well as other pharmacological therapies for inflammatory conditions. The latest version of relevant clinical guidelines is provided, and self-assessment questions (with answers available on the publisher's website) have been refined.

Our sincerest thanks go to Scion Publishing, to Jonathan Ray for his persistent but gentle nudges that have been inspirational reminders to the authors, to Jonathan's team for their guidance and help throughout the process, and to my many colleagues in Rheumatology who have ungrudgingly provided advice in their specialist areas. I hope that the second edition is received with the same warmth as before.

Ash Samanta
Emeritus Consultant Rheumatologist,
University of Leicester

Preface to the first edition

In my experience of teaching rheumatology at undergraduate (and postgraduate) level for over thirty years, there is one consistent response that I have come across from medical students. This is a general fear of rheumatology. The reason many students regard rheumatology as mysterious and arcane is because of a lack of understanding about what rheumatology covers, as well as a somewhat fuzzy knowledge of the various conditions that are encompassed within rheumatology.

Some years ago I thought it might be helpful for medical students (at the University of Leicester) if I put together what I termed 'revision notes' for rheumatology. I would often encourage students to offer any suggestions for change but the reality was that no-one ever did. A couple of years ago, two bright young medical students, Ahmad Al-Sukaini and Mohsin Azam (who are co-authors of this text) approached me after one of my lectures and came up with a number of ideas, and the revision notes were updated in due course. They also suggested putting together a short book that would be more comprehensive than just brief notes, and that would flag key issues in rheumatology for undergraduate medical students. Their enthusiasm, effort and assistance are to be strongly commended.

According to surveys we carried out at the University of Leicester, students wholeheartedly agreed that a rheumatology 'guide' would be of benefit to them and to junior doctors. Their preference was to use bullet point formatting and an approach that would be succinct and highly focused, as opposed to the more conventional paragraphs and narrative writing. We have also used a wide range of pedagogic features, including summary tables, illustrations and mnemonics throughout. Furthermore, the size of the book was important – it had to be one that could be carried around easily. To test student knowledge and reinforce learning, questions were devised within the framework used by examiners. Single Best Answer (SBA) and Extended Matching Questions (EMQs) are increasingly being utilized by medical school examiners to explore understanding of a topic and it is essential that students familiarize themselves with these types of question. The questions, together with their answers, can be found online, as mentioned at the end of the Contents.

We took up this challenge and have put together this text with the aim of covering rheumatology in a clear and concise manner. The content thoroughly encompasses the current medical school curriculum in the UK and we hope that this text will be highly beneficial to medical students for furthering their knowledge, as well as a revision guide for undergraduate examination purposes. We also hope that it will assist newly qualified junior doctors and serve as a quick reference guide for clinics and ward-based work. The concise and coherent format of this book is likely to appeal to other healthcare professionals who require a working knowledge of rheumatology.

Finally, I would say that this text is not intended to replace any of the standard erudite text books in rheumatology that have already been published. It is designed to focus the mind, provide concise guidance, and encourage further exploration of rheumatology.

Dr Ash Samanta
Consultant Rheumatologist, University of Leicester
January 2014

Acknowledgments

We would like to place on record our sincere gratitude to the team at Scion Publishing Ltd, particularly Dr Jonathan Ray and Ms Clare Boomer, for their great support, encouragement and patience.

Please refer to the Appendix for acknowledgment to the copyright holders of the many images in the book.

Dedications

To my son Yasin and daughter Elanur – you bring so much joy and warmth into my life. M.A.

For my family, and the friends who create 'home'. G.S.

For my 'long-suffering' family. A.S.

Abbreviations

ACA	anti-centromere antibody
ACE	angiotension-converting enzyme
ACR	American College of Rheumatology
ALP	alkaline phosphatase
ANA	antinuclear antibodies
ANCA	antineutrophil cytoplasmic antibodies
APS	antiphospholipid syndrome
ARF	acute renal failure
AS	ankylosing spondylitis
AxSpA	axial spondyloarthropathies
BMD	bone mineral density
BMI	body mass index
BP	blood pressure
CBT	cognitive behavioural therapy
CCF	congestive cardiac failure
CCP	cyclic citrullinated peptide
CK	creatine kinase
CNS	central nervous system
CPPD	calcium pyrophosphate disease
CRP	C-reactive protein
CSS	Churg–Strauss syndrome
CT	computerized tomography
CVE	cerebrovascular event
CVS	cardiovascular system
CXR	chest X-ray
DAS	Disease Activity Score
DEXA	dual-energy X-ray absorptiometry
DIP	distal interphalangeal
DM	dermatomyositis
DMARD	disease-modifying antirheumatic drug
DNA	deoxyribonucleic acid
DVT	deep vein thrombosis
ECG	electrocardiogram
EDTA	ethylenediaminetetraacetic acid
EMG	electromyography
ERA	endothelin-1 receptor antagonists
ESR	erythrocyte sedimentation rate
EULAR	European Alliance of Associations for Rheumatology
FBC	full blood count
FDG	fluorodeoxyglucose
FRAX	Fracture Risk Assessment Tool
FSH	follicle-stimulating hormone
GBM	glomerular basement disease
GCA	giant cell arteritis
GCS	glucocorticosteroid
GI	gastrointestinal
GORD	gastro-oesophageal reflux disease
GPA	granulomatosis with polyangiitis
GU	genitourinary
HAART	highly active antiretroviral treatment
Hb	haemoglobin
HBV	hepatitis B virus
HLA	human leucocyte antigen
HRT	hormone replacement therapy
HSP	Henoch–Schönlein purpura
IBD	inflammatory bowel disease
IHD	ischaemic heart disease
IL	interleukin
ILAR	International League of Associations for Rheumatology
IV	intravenous
JIA	juvenile idiopathic arthritis
JRA	juvenile rheumatoid arthritis
LDH	lactate dehydrogenase
LFT	liver function test
MAS	macrophage activation syndrome
MCP	metacarpophalangeal
MCTD	mixed connective tissue disease
ME/CFS	myalgic encephalomyelitis / chronic fatigue syndrome
MI	myocardial infarction
MMF	mycophenolate mofetil
MMP	metalloprotease

MPA	microscopic polyangiitis
MRI	magnetic resonance imaging
MSK	musculoskeletal
MSU	monosodium urate
MTP	metatarso-phalangeal
NICE	National Institute for Health and Care Excellence
NSAID	non-steroidal anti-inflammatory drug
OA	osteoarthritis
PAN	polyarteritis nodosa
PCV	packed cell volume
PDE	phosphodiesterase
PE	pulmonary embolism
PIP	proximal interphalangeal
PM	polymyositis
PMR	polymyalgia rheumatica
PPI	proton pump inhibitor
PsA	psoriatic arthritis
PTH	parathyroid hormone
RA	rheumatoid arthritis
ReA	reactive arthritis
RF	rheumatoid factor
RFT	renal function test
ROS	reactive oxygen species
SCAR	severe cutaneous adverse reaction
SI	sacroiliac
SLE	systemic lupus erythematosus
SpA	spondyloarthropathy
SS	Sjögren's syndrome
SSc	systemic sclerosis
SUA	serum uric acid
TB	tuberculosis
TFT	thyroid function test
TNF	tumour necrosis factor
USS	ultrasound scan
UTI	urinary tract infection
VTE	venous thromboembolism
WCC	white cell count
WG	Wegener's granulomatosis
WHO	World Health Organization
XOi	xanthine oxidase inhibitor

Chapter 1

Introduction

What is rheumatology?

Rheumatology is a multidisciplinary branch of medicine that encompasses the investigation, diagnosis and management of patients with arthritis and other musculoskeletal conditions. This includes many disorders affecting joints, bones, muscles and soft tissues. A significant number of musculoskeletal conditions also affect other organ systems and occur as part of a systemic autoimmune disease. The main rheumatological disorders are summarized in *Fig. 1.1* and will be covered in significant depth.

The rheumatology multidisciplinary team (MDT) consists of a variety of disciplines that work together with the aim of providing optimal care to sufferers via a holistic approach (*Fig. 1.2*). The team consists of many healthcare professionals including consultant rheumatologists, general practitioners (GPs), occupational therapists, orthopaedic surgeons, physiotherapists, psychiatrists, specialist nurses and many more.

Rheumatologists are specialists who deal with a wide range of rheumatic diseases. They assess overall function, including physical and mental wellbeing and level of independence. They also manage results of advanced imaging and lab tests, treatment options and the need for further assessment and management, such as referrals to other healthcare providers.

Outline of the book

Chapter 2

For each condition the following will be covered:

- ***Pathophysiology***: the information surrounding the pathophysiology of rheumatology disorders is constantly evolving and there is still so much that remains to be understood. Up-to-date resources were used with the intention of keeping this section simple and concise and not overlooking the clinical aspects of rheumatology!
- ***Epidemiology and risk factors***: attention has been paid to the incidence / prevalence of the rheumatology disorders so that students are aware of the very common, less common and rare disorders. Where possible, risk factors are arranged in a descending order of importance via a simple to follow table, to highlight the most important risk factors for students to learn.
- ***Clinical features***: a variety of pedagogical features such as X-rays, photographs and illustrations have been used, as well as **red flags** indicated by (flag icon), and mnemonics in **green**. Red flags or alarm systems refer to symptoms which are suggestive of significant pathology and should therefore not be missed or neglected. These devices are aimed at enabling students to have a greater understanding of the features to look out for and also as an aid to information retention.
- ***Diagnosis and investigations***: this element is centred on the diagnostic pathway – history taking, physical examination, investigations and possible differential diagnoses. It is conveyed in an easy to follow box format. Wherever relevant, up-to-date clinical guidelines, including those from the National Institute for Health and Care Excellence (NICE), the European Alliance of Associations for Rheumatology (EULAR) and the American College of Rheumatology (ACR), were utilized. *Chapter 4* has also been created specifically for investigations, to provide further detail of the various tests performed in rheumatology.

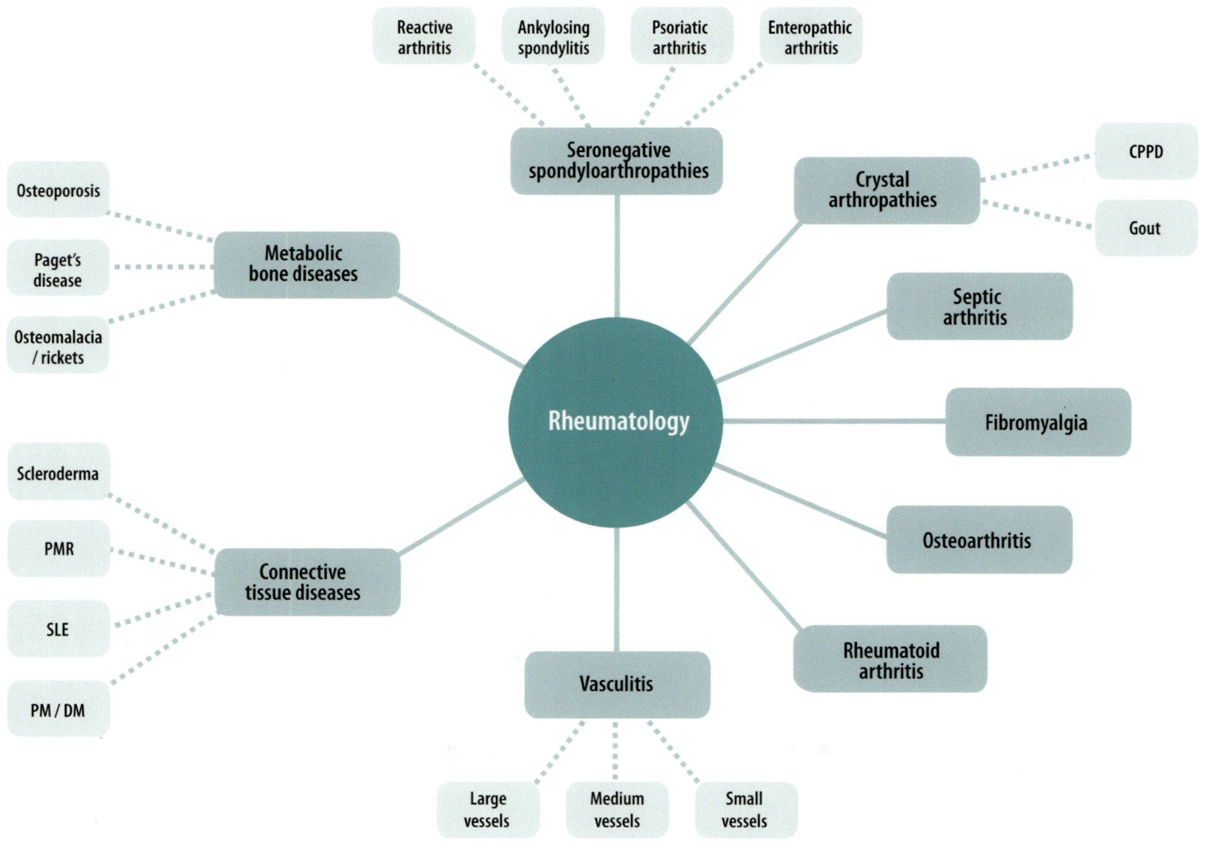

Fig. 1.1: An outline of the main rheumatological disorders.

- ***Management***: this part also utilizes clinical guidelines. Flowcharts, tables and diagrams are used to convey information more effectively and render it more memorable. *Chapter 5* covers the main pharmacological agents of rheumatology in further detail.
- ***OSCE tip / rapid diagnosis / clinical fact box:*** wherever applicable, extra information is provided in the form of tips for the OSCE examination, empirical diagnostic features to form a 'rapid diagnosis' and important clinical facts for students to be aware of.

Self-assessment questions conclude each specific condition section. These are designed for students to check that they have understood and grasped the material.

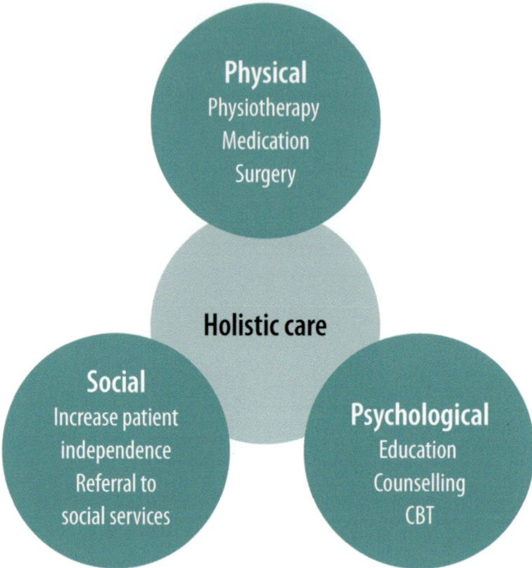

Fig. 1.2: An MDT holistic approach outline to rheumatology.

Chapter 3

This chapter consists of two important and common conditions in rheumatology which present during early life: vitamin D deficiency including both rickets and osteomalacia and juvenile idiopathic arthritis. The same longitudinal format is used as above.

Chapter 4

It may be advisable to read this before embarking on the main rheumatological conditions text (*Chapter 2*), as it provides a basic understanding of the three principal investigations used in rheumatology to reach a definitive diagnosis: blood tests, imaging and synovial fluid analysis.

Chapter 5

This should be used as a cross-reference with *Chapter 2*, in order for students to gain a deeper understanding of the way in which pharmacological agents work, as well as the side-effects and contraindications. It provides information about commonly used agents including analgesics, corticosteroids, osteoporosis agents, DMARDs and biological agents. This section also includes '**DO**' and '**DO NOT**' boxes so that students are aware of the essentials and common pitfalls, respectively, when prescribing pharmacological agents.

Chapter 6

This focuses on the key points of history taking and performing clinical examinations, with particular emphasis on the GALS and hand examination, so that students have a thorough structure to follow and therefore do not panic when it comes to the dreaded OSCE examinations!

Additional questions in the form of single best answer questions (SBAs) and extended matching questions (EMQs) have been made available online as a free resource to complement the material in the book. To access the questions and answers, click on the Resources tab at www.scionpublishing.com/Rheum2.

Chapter 2

Specific conditions

2.1	Rheumatoid arthritis	8
2.2	Osteoarthritis	15
2.3	Septic arthritis	20
	Introduction to spondyloarthropathies	24
2.4	Psoriatic arthritis	25
2.5	Ankylosing spondylitis	30
2.6	Reactive arthritis	35
2.7	Gout	39
2.8	Calcium pyrophosphate disease	44
2.9	Vasculitis	47
2.10	Giant cell arteritis	55
2.11	Polymyalgia rheumatica	59
2.12	Systemic lupus erythematosus	62
2.13	Polymyositis and dermatomyositis	69
2.14	Sjögren's syndrome	74
2.15	Scleroderma	78
2.16	Fibromyalgia	84
2.17	Osteoporosis	88
2.18	Paget's disease	93

2.1 Rheumatoid arthritis

Rheumatoid arthritis (RA) is a **chronic systemic inflammatory** disorder which primarily affects joints that are lined with **synovium**. It is typically characterized by a **symmetrical**, occasionally **deforming**, **peripheral polyarthritis**. Because it is a **systemic disease**, it can also affect the whole body, including the heart, lungs and eyes. Cardiovascular disease is the leading cause of mortality in RA.

Pathophysiology

- The actual cause of RA is not entirely understood.
- It is likely that **genetically susceptible** individuals, e.g. HLA-DRB1 carriers, are exposed to an environmental antigen or factors (such as tobacco smoke, occupational dust) resulting in self-stimulation of the immune system **(autoimmunity)**.
- The immune response cross-reacts with the **host tissue (synovial membrane)** resulting in **inflammation** of the **synovial membrane (synovitis)** that lines **joints** and **tendon sheaths**. This gives rise to **synovial hypertrophy**.
- **T-cells** seem to be the most important mediators of the disease. They stimulate the immune system via the release of a variety of **inflammatory cytokines**, most importantly **TNF-α**, **IL-1**, **IL-17**, and **IL-6**, resulting in a **pro-inflammatory state** (*Fig. 2.1.1*). There may also be a deficit in the regulation or apoptosis of T-cells, contributing to pathogenesis.
- **Synovial macrophages, fibroblasts and autoreactive B-cells** are the drivers of RA and produce autoantibodies (**rheumatoid factor** and **anti-citrullinated protein antibodies**) (**RF** and **anti-CCP**). They are the primary generators of TNF-α and other inflammatory cytokines.
- This process can ultimately lead to **cartilage damage** and **bone destruction** by activating osteoclasts, resulting in periarticular osteopenia, bone erosions, and generalized osteoporosis.
- Bone formation is also reduced as **osteoblast** maturation is suppressed by **TNF-α**.

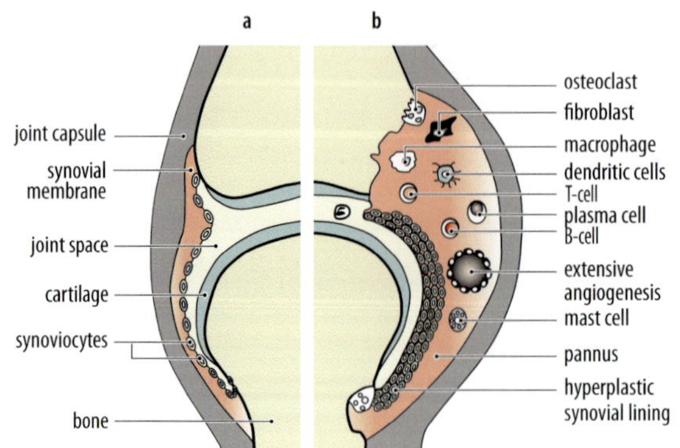

Fig. 2.1.1: (a) Normal healthy joint with thin synovial membrane and **(b)** an RA joint. Various inflammatory cells, such as T-cells, macrophages and plasma cells, infiltrate the synovial membrane to make it hyperplastic. Ultimately it develops into a 'pannus' which migrates onto and into articular cartilage and underlying bone.

Epidemiology and risk factors

- **Prevalence**: there are approximately 680 000 people with RA in the UK (~1%).
- **Incidence**: approximately 1.5 men and 3.6 women are diagnosed with RA per 10 000 people per year in the UK.
- Certain risk factors have been linked to RA (*Table 2.1.1*).

Table 2.1.1: Risk factors for RA	
Gender	• **Before menopause**, RA is **3 times** more common in **women** than men; after menopause the distribution is similar.
Age	• Rheumatoid arthritis can affect any age group, but the age of onset is often **30–50 years**.
Familial	• Estimated to account for **60%** of disease susceptibility.
Genetic	• There are strong associations between **HLA-DR4 and HLA-DR1** and RA, which may be **familial or non-familial (sporadic)**.
Environmental factors	• **Smoking (2.5–3.5× risk)**, infection (there may be a relationship with EBV or *P. gingivalis*), diet, microbiome and hormonal.

Clinical features

The **S** factor:

1. **Stiffness** in the morning typically >1 hour
2. **Symmetrical** joint pain
3. **Swollen joints** (polyarthritis)
4. **Small joints** of the hand, feet and wrist (mainly affected)
5. **Sex**: female:male ratio is 3:1
6. **Speed: quick onset** over weeks to **months**
7. **Specific signs for the hand**:
   a. ***Early***: swollen metacarpophalangeal (MCP), proximal interphalangeal (PIP), wrist or metatarso-phalangeal (MTP) joints.
   b. ***Later*** (*Fig. 2.1.2a*): **boutonnière deformity** (flexion of the PIP and hyperextension of the distal interphalangeal (DIP) joints), **swan neck deformity** (hyperextension of PIP and flexion of DIP joints), **Z-thumb** (hyperextension of the interphalangeal joint, and fixed flexion and subluxation of the MCP joint) and **ulnar deviation** (subluxation of proximal phalanges towards the ulnar side).
8. **Several extra-articular manifestations** (*Fig. 2.1.3*).

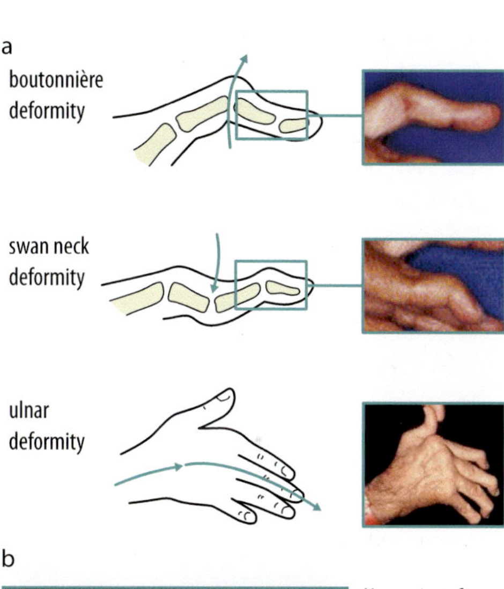

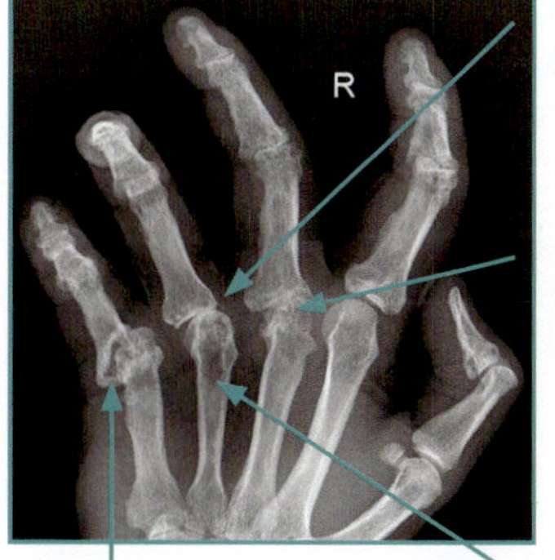

Fig. 2.1.2: **(a)** Late specific signs of RA; **(b)** Late X-ray features of RA.

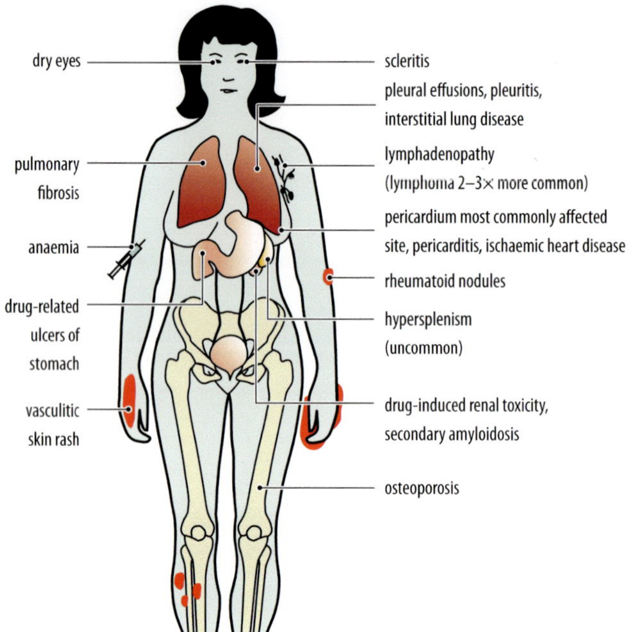

Fig. 2.1.3: The extra-articular manifestations of the disease can occur at any age after onset and occur more commonly in males, despite RA being more common in females. Extra-articular organs may involve the skin, eyes, heart, lungs and kidneys.

OSCE tips: RA vs OA clinical features!

- **RA** usually presents symmetrically, osteoarthritis (**OA**) usually presents with asymmetrical joint pain
- **RA** morning stiffness usually >1 hour, **OA** stiffness usually <30 minutes
- **OA** is worse on movement, **RA** is not
- **RA** is more likely to involve the distal small joints (MCP, PIP and MTP), whereas **OA** is likely to affect larger joints (hip, knee, shoulder)
- Common age of onset for **RA** is 20–40 years and >50 years for **OA**
- **RA** onset is relatively rapid (weeks to months), **OA** typically years
- **RA** presents with systemic symptoms, **OA** doesn't
- **RA** tends to be worse in the morning; **OA** is worse after activities, especially towards the end of the day

Diagnosis and investigations (see *Table 2.1.2*)

All people suspected of having RA should be referred for specialist assessment.

	Diagnosis	Prognostic indicators
Hx	• Pain duration (usually ≥6 weeks), morning stiffness >1 hour	• Activity limitations, comorbidities, risk factors such as smoking and family history
Ex	• ≥3 swollen tender joints, symmetrical joint involvement, subcutaneous nodules	• Extra-articular manifestations (*Fig. 2.1.3*)
Ix	• ↑ **Serum rheumatoid factor (RF)** • ↑ **Anti-cyclic citrullinated peptide antibodies (anti-CCP)** • ↑ **Erythrocyte sedimentation rate (ESR) / C-reactive protein (CRP)** **Note:** *RF has ↑ sensitivity and ↓ specificity; anti-CCP has ↑ specificity and ↓ sensitivity*	• **Full blood count**: ↑ platelet count, ↑ serum ferritin, anaemia of chronic disease • **Renal and liver function tests** • **X-ray**: chest, hands (*Fig. 2.1.2b*) and feet • **MRI**: identify synovitis early • **Ultrasound**: joint effusion, Baker's cysts and synovial swelling/hypertrophy
DDx	• Psoriatic arthritis • Connective tissue disease, e.g. systemic lupus erythematosus (SLE)	• Reactive arthritis • Polymyalgia rheumatica

Table 2.1.2: The 2010 American College of Rheumatology (ACR) and the European Alliance of Associations for Rheumatology (EULAR) criteria

The most recent criteria for the diagnosis of RA are the 2010 ACR and the EULAR criteria. A total score of ≥6 is diagnostic of RA.	Score
A. Joint involvement:	
1 large joint	0
2–10 large joints	1
1–3 small joints (with or without involvement of large joints)	2
4–10 small joints (with or without involvement of large joints)	3
B. Serology:	
Negative RF and negative anti-CCP	0
Low-positive RF or low-positive anti-CCP	2
High-positive RF or high-positive anti-CCP	3
C. Acute phase reactants:	
Normal CRP and normal ESR	0
Abnormal CRP or abnormal ESR	1
D. Duration of symptoms:	
<6 weeks	0
≥6 weeks	1

Note: The 2010 EULAR and ACR criteria replaced the 1987 ACR criteria as they focus on features at an earlier stage of the disease that are associated with persistent and/or erosive disease, rather than defining the disease by its late-stage features. As a result, this refocuses attention on the important need for earlier diagnosis and therefore earlier treatment.

Management

The aim of management in RA is to reduce / slow the joint inflammation and disease progression to maintain the patient's lifestyle. Early use of **disease-modifying antirheumatic drugs (DMARDs)** and **biological agents** improves the long-term outcome of the disease. Treatment should be started **within 3 months** of symptom onset, based on NICE NG100 (2018, updated 2020).

- Refer urgently to a **rheumatologist**, in order to prevent irreversible destruction of joint(s) if:
  - the **small joints of the hand and feet** are affected
  - more than one joint is affected
  - there has been a delay of 3 months or longer between the onset of symptoms and seeking medical advice.
- Consider NSAID and PPI in the interim.
- Specialists usually start with a conventional DMARD **(cDMARD)** monotherapy and short-term **corticosteroids** (bridging if appropriate).
- Emphasis should be placed on reaching a clinical effective dose rather than on the choice of DMARD.
- If the disease is severe and a combination of **cDMARDs** have not been sufficient, biologic DMARDs (**bDMARDs**) may be offered.
- The disease activity of RA should be monitored by measuring **CRP** and the **DAS28 score** (*Box 2.1.1*). The aim is to reduce the **DAS28 score below 3**. However, DAS28 score may be subjective and is highly examiner-dependent.
- Patient-driven composite tools such as **RAPID3** can also be used as they are more time-efficient and may provide a more reliable measurement of change over time.
- DMARDs need monitoring (generally every 3 months once stable) and frequently include: FBC, LFT and U & E.

Non-pharmacological management

- Encourage regular exercise: aerobic activities, flexibility and muscle strength exercises, **core stability exercise**, **balance rehabilitation**, promotion of lifestyle physical activity, smoking cessation, healthy balanced diet.
- People with RA should have access to a **multidisciplinary team** such as **specialist nurses**, **physiotherapists**, **occupational therapists** and **podiatrists**.

Pharmacological: see *Table 2.1.3*

Surgery:

- Consider the following for surgical opinion if they do not respond to non-surgical management:
  - **Persistent pain** due to joint damage or other identifiable soft tissue cause
  - **Worsening joint function**
  - **Progressive deformity**
  - **Persistent localized synovitis**.

Table 2.1.3: Pharmacological management of rheumatoid arthritis

cDMARDs	• Are **first-line** • Early DMARD treatment (ideally within 3 months from symptom onset) is associated with better long-term prognosis • **Methotrexate**, **sulfasalazine**, **leflunomide** and **hydroxychloroquine** are the most commonly used • NICE recommends a combination of DMARDs, including methotrexate and at least one other DMARD, plus short-term glucocorticoids (if not contraindicated)
Corticosteroids	• Rapid reduction in **symptom onset** and **inflammation** • Can be given via **intra-muscular**, **intra-articular** and **oral routes** • NICE recommends a combination of DMARD ± a short course of bridging prednisolone
NSAIDs	For **symptomatic relief** and also to **reduce inflammation**, e.g. **ibuprofen**, **naproxen**, **diclofenac**
Biological agents (bDMARDs) (TNF-α inhibitors, B-cell blockers, and anti-IL-1 & IL-6 agents). Indications: after the failure of 2 conventional non-biological DMARDs. Failure is measured objectively using DAS28 (indicated by a score >5.1)	
TNF-α inhibitors	• Usually indicated when there is an inadequate response to at least 2 DMARDs (including methotrexate) • Block the pivotal action of TNF-α, a key cytokine in the pathogenesis of RA • Include **infliximab**, **adalimumab** and **etanercept** • Very **expensive** and used in **severe cases (high DAS28 score)** • Should normally be used in combination with methotrexate • Risks include reactivation of tuberculosis (TB)
B-cell blockers	• **Rituximab** is a **monoclonal antibody** • It works by targeting the **B-cell surface marker**, **CD-20** • It is given via IV infusions 2 weeks apart • A combination of **rituximab** and **methotrexate** is recommended as an option for the treatment of adults with RA who are intolerant of other DMARDs or whose response to them is inadequate
Anti IL-1 & IL-6 agents	• Like TNF- α, IL-1 and IL-6 are pro-inflammatory cytokines which are heavily involved in the disease process • **Anakinra** is an **IL-1 receptor antagonist** • **Tocilizumab** is an **anti-IL-6 receptor monoclonal antibody** • On the balance of its clinical benefits and cost-effectiveness, anakinra is not recommended for the treatment of rheumatoid arthritis
JAK inhibitors	• **Tofacitinib** and **baricitinib** are **JAK inhibitors** • Block cytokines via inhibition of **Janus kinases** • Targeted synthetic DMARDs that can be given in tablet form • Risk of thrombotic events, and infection (immunosuppression)

- Surgical procedures may include:
  - **Joint prosthesis**: **hip** and **knee**
  - **Arthroscopy**: remove abnormal synovium, cartilage and eroded bone
  - **Tendon reconstruction**: restore function when tendon ruptured.

Box 2.1.1: The Disease Activity Score (DAS)28

- It assesses **tenderness and swelling at 28 joints** (see *Fig. 2.1.4*), **ESR**, and patients' **self-reported symptom** severity, to calculate a disease activity score.
  DAS28 score of:
  >5.1 = high disease activity
  3.2–5.1 = moderate disease activity
  <3.2 = low disease activity
  <2.6 = remission
- ***A decrease in DAS28 score by***:
  0.6 points or less = poor response
  >1.2 points = moderate or good response
  (depending on whether an individual's DAS28 score at the end point is above or below 3.2, respectively)

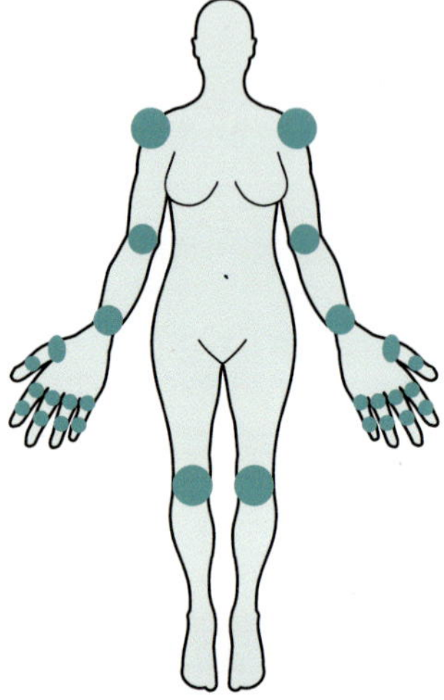

Fig. 2.1.4: The 28 joints (MCPs, PIPs, wrists, elbows, shoulders and knees) that are examined in calculating DAS28.

Self-assessment

A 45 year old woman complains of symmetrical pain and swelling of her MCP joints. You think that a diagnosis of RA is likely.

1. What specific questions would you like to ask her?
2. Name two hand deformities that can be caused by RA.
3. What blood tests would you initially perform, and what might they show?
4. Name four extra-articular manifestations of RA.
5. The blood tests confirm a diagnosis of RA. Which group of pharmacological agents would be most appropriate in preventing disease progression? Name the most used drug in this group and its main side-effects.
6. Name two ways of monitoring response to treatment.

Answers to self-assessment questions are to be found on the Resources tab at www.scionpublishing.com/Rheum2.

2.2 Osteoarthritis

Osteoarthritis (OA) is the **most common form of arthritis** and is a major cause of **impaired mobility.** It is a chronic condition which occurs when damage triggers repair processes resulting in **cartilage damage** and **joint space narrowing** leading to **pain**, **functional limitation** and **impaired quality of life.** It can affect any joint but the **hip**, **knee**, **lumbar** or **cervical spine**, and **wrist joints** are most commonly affected.

Pathophysiology

- OA is viewed as a **metabolically dynamic process** where there is an imbalance between joint breakdown and sufficient repair process.
- Normal joint articulating cartilage, **hyaline cartilage**, undergoes turnover in which 'worn out' collagen and other matrix components are degraded and replaced by **chondrocyte cells**.
- Both **genetic and environmental** factors can stimulate **apoptosis** of chondrocytes, disrupting the normal repair mechanism and thereby causing cartilage damage, or **hypertrophy and cluster** of the chondrocytes, increasing production of enzymes, which degrade the matrix and 'use up' **proteoglycans**. The cartilage swells due to the breakdown of **proteoglycans**, making it more vulnerable to damage.
- Certain **cytokines** (e.g. **IL-1** and **TNF-α**) and **protease enzymes** (e.g. **metalloproteinase**) increase in the cartilage, which triggers osteoarthritic changes through direct cartilage damage. They activate **osteoblasts** and **osteoclasts**.
- Eventually, cartilage destruction exposes underlying bone, resulting in abnormal **subchondral bone growth (subchondral sclerosis)**, **osteophytes** and **bone cysts** (*Fig. 2.2.1*).
- In OA, the synovium becomes inflamed and swells, which leads to synovial cell proliferation. This may be accentuated by **calcium phosphate** and **calcium pyrophosphate dihydrate crystals** which are released by the cartilage. This **increases** intra-articular pressure and stimulates **nociceptors (pain).** This may overlap with pseudogout (*Sec. 2.8*).
- The articular capsule may become fibrotic which may lead to pathological weakness in the bridge of the joint and surrounding muscles.

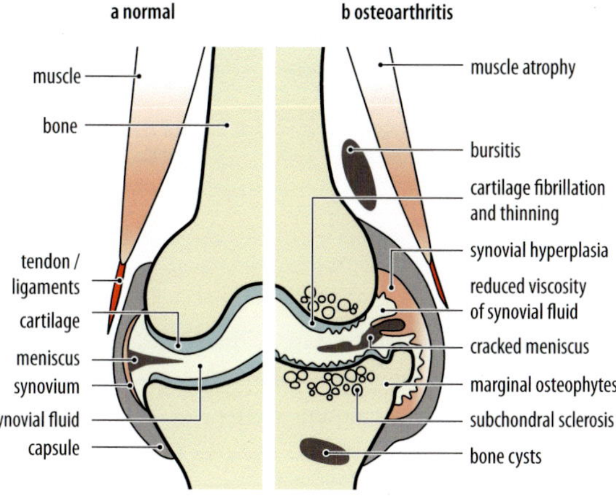

Fig. 2.2.1: (a) Normal joint **(b)** OA joint.

Epidemiology and risk factors

- Worldwide estimates indicate that there are approximately 429 people per 100 000 with OA.
- Approximately a third of women and nearly a quarter of men aged 45–64 have sought treatment for OA in the UK.

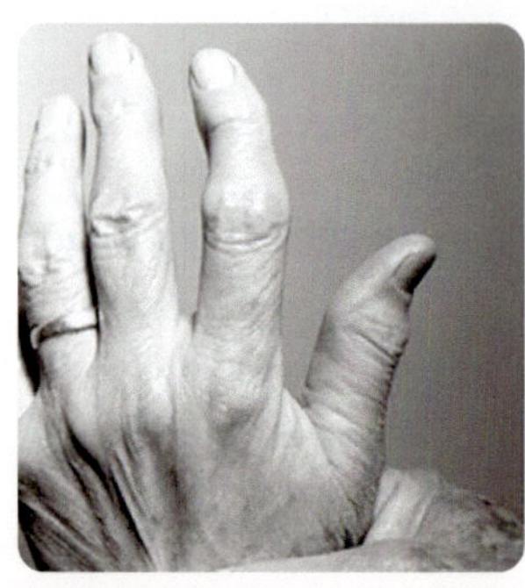

Fig. 2.2.2: Bony enlargements of the DIP joints (Heberden's nodes) and PIP joints (Bouchard's nodes) due to osteophyte formation.

Table 2.2.1: Risk factors for OA

Systemic risk factors		**Mechanical risk factors**	
Age	• Risk increases with age; partly due to age-related changes such as ligament laxity (ligaments are joint protectors). There is a reduction in normal repair response.	**Obesity**	• Places mechanical stress on joint cartilage.
Gender	• Polyarticular OA is more common in women. • A high prevalence in post-menopausal women suggests a role for sex hormones.	**Injury**	• Ligament damage or fractures can lead to abnormal stress on joint cartilage.
		Joint damage	• Joint damage due to underlying disease, e.g. RA, Paget's disease, varus and valgus deformity or trauma (secondary OA).
Family history	• 40–60% of 'common OA' is thought to have a hereditary component. This is joint-specific.	**Joint site**	• Weight-bearing joints are at higher risk.
Bone density	• ↑ bone density e.g. Paget's disease ↑ risk of OA. • ↓ bone density e.g. osteoporosis ↓ risk of OA.	**Occupation**	• Cleaners have ↑ risk of hip, knee and shoulder OA. • Hairdressers have ↑ risk of hand OA. • Farmers have ↑ risk of hip OA.

Clinical features

- Clinical features depend on the joint sites affected (*Table 2.2.2*).

  Symptoms: **joint pain** – usually gradual onset, worse on movement, load bearing and at the end of the day, **joint stiffness** – in the morning or after rest for <30 minutes, **reduced joint function** and **joint instability**.

  Signs: **periarticular tenderness**, **crepitus**, ↓ range of movement, **muscle wasting**, **joint deformity** and **instability**, squaring of the thumb, swelling of the hands (**Bouchard's nodes** and **Heberden's nodes**; *Fig. 2.2.2*), mild **synovitis** and **effusion**.

Table 2.2.2: American College of Rheumatology (ACR) criteria for hand, hip and knee OA	
Nodal OA	Nodal OA or primary generalized OA commonly affects post-menopausal women. There is hand pain, aching, or stiffness for most days of the prior month. Heberden's and Bouchard's nodes in ≥2 joints are characteristic of nodal OA. EULAR has released classification criteria for hand OA based on the same criteria, with the addition of age, number of joints with osteophytes, and X-ray findings.
Hip OA	Hip pain for most days of the prior month. Categorized largely radiographically: femoral and/or acetabular osteophytes and radiograph hip joint-space narrowing.
Knee OA	Commonly presents in obese women ≥38 years of age. There is knee pain for most days of the prior month, crepitus on movement, morning stiffness ≤30 minutes and bony enlargement of the knee on examination.

Diagnosis and investigations

Hx

- **Joint pain** (worsened by exercise & relieved by rest) and **stiffness** (morning / after rest).
- **Reduced joint function** and **joint instability**.
- Ask about **risk factors** e.g. family history and trauma.

Ex

- **Look** → pain on movement, muscle wasting and limp/antalgic gait.
- **Feel** → periarticular tenderness, swelling of joints, mild synovitis and effusion, and absence of systemic features, e.g. fever.
- **Move** → pain on movement, ↓ range of movement, joint deformity, joint instability and crepitus.

Ix

- **Blood tests**: ESR and CRP are usually normal, RF and anti-CCP negative.
- **Joint aspiration**: sterile, straw-coloured, viscous fluid; white cell count (WCC) may be slightly elevated.
- **X-ray ('LOSS')**: **Loss of joint space**, **Osteophytes**, **Subchondral sclerosis**, **Subchondral cysts** (*Figs 2.2.3* and *2.2.4*). This also helps with grading the severity of OA.
- **MRI**: can demonstrate early thinning of cartilage.
- **Arthroscopy**: cartilage loss and erosion.

DDx

Large joint involvement:

- Monoarticular inflammatory arthropathy
- Chronic infection e.g. tuberculosis
- Calcium pyrophosphate disease (CPPD) (if knee is involved)

Small polyarticular joint involvement:

- RA

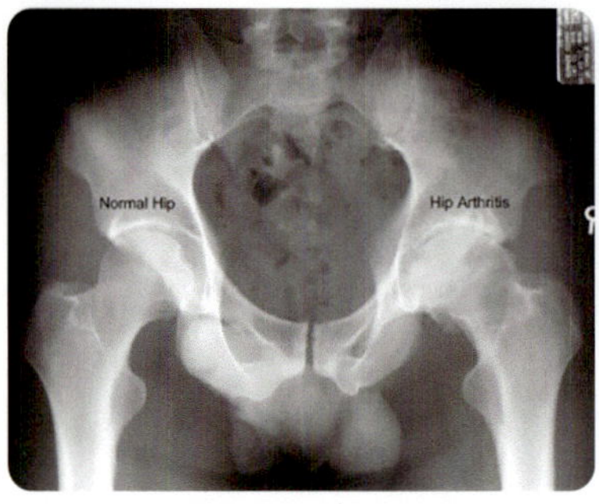

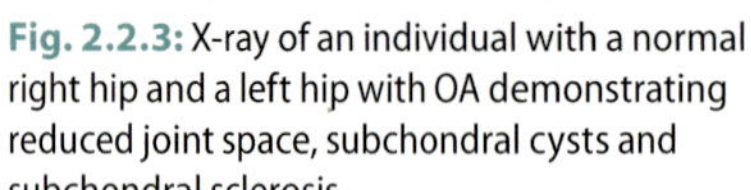

Fig. 2.2.3: X-ray of an individual with a normal right hip and a left hip with OA demonstrating reduced joint space, subchondral cysts and subchondral sclerosis.

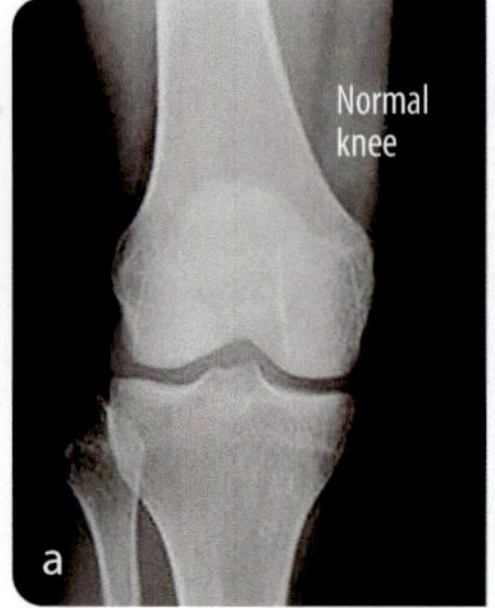

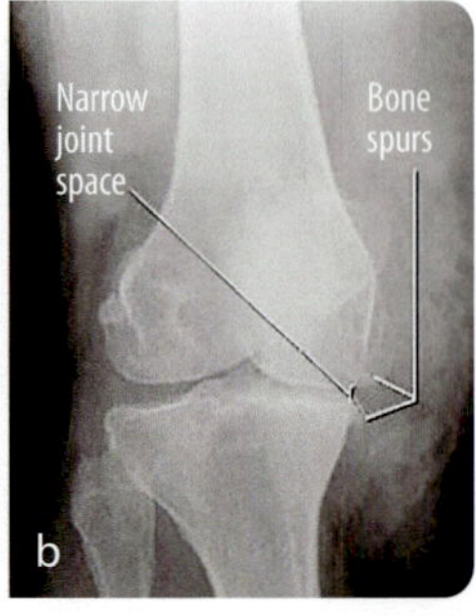

Fig. 2.2.4: X-ray of **(a)** a normal joint and **(b)** an osteoarthritic knee which shows reduced joint space and bony spurs (osteophytes).

OSCE tips: Specific questions to ask someone with suspected OA

- **Presenting complaint** → Joint pain worse on exercise or after rest? Is there morning stiffness? If so, for how long? Reduced joint function and stability? Weight-bearing joint(s)? Particular joint(s) that is 'overused'?
- **Predisposing factors** → e.g. history of trauma?
- **Past medical history** → Secondary causes e.g. RA and Paget's disease?
- **Family history** → Family history of OA?
- **Social history** → Current/previous occupation? How are their symptoms impacting them?

Management (NICE guidelines, 2022)

- Management of OA includes non-pharmacological management (*Table 2.2.3*), pharmacological pain relief (*Fig. 2.2.5*) and surgical intervention.

Table 2.2.3: Non-pharmacological management of OA

Education and advice	Education, advice and access to information are core treatments which should be offered to everyone with OA (www.versusarthritis.org). Self-management programmes should be encouraged.
Exercise	Exercise should be a core treatment for people with OA and should consist of local muscle strengthening and general aerobic fitness.
Weight loss	Should be a core treatment for OA individuals who are obese or overweight. Behaviour change techniques should be used.
Aids and devices	Advice on appropriate footwear should be given as part of core treatment for people with lower limb OA. In some cases people with biomechanical joint pain or instability may be considered for bracing / joint supports / insoles / walking sticks / frames if exercise is ineffective.

Table 2.2.3: Non-pharmacological management of OA *(continued)*	
Physiotherapy and occupational therapy	Manual joint manipulation may be useful for some individuals with hip and knee OA. Advice should be given on modifiable work-related factors. Occupational therapy assessment for any adjustments at work or in the home.
Psychosocial support	Motivational coaching, pain coping and goal setting.

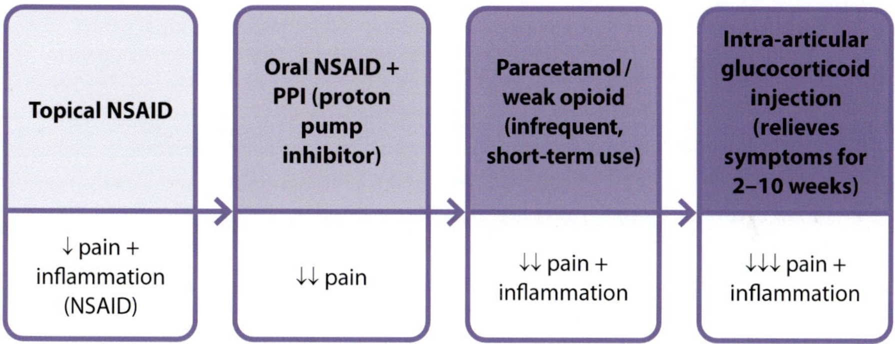

Fig. 2.2.5: Pharmacological management of OA.

- Surgical intervention is indicated when joint symptoms have a substantial impact on the patient's quality of life and medical management has failed. Scoring tools, age, gender and BMI should not be used to exclude patients from surgery.
  - **Replacement of joint** – the most common operations are to replace hip, knee, and base of thumb joints. The ankle joint can be fused or replaced.
  - **Arthroscopy lavage and debridement are not recommended as per current evidence-based guidance** (https://doi.org/10.1136/bjsports-2017-j1982rep) (2018).

Self-assessment

A 68 year old female has been complaining of bilateral hip pain for the last 6 weeks. An X-ray is then performed (*Fig. 2.2.6*).

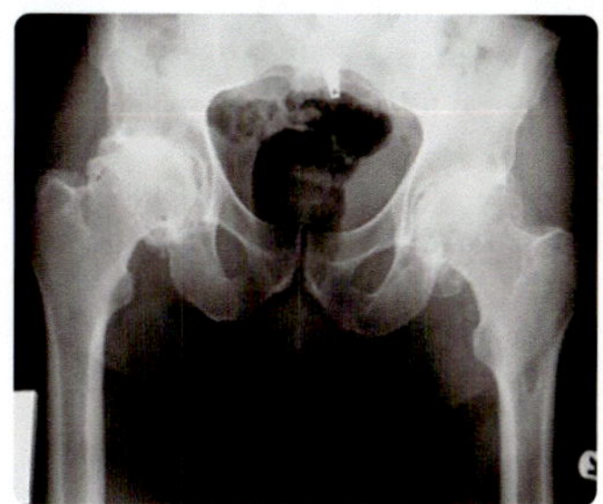

Fig. 2.2.6: X-ray of pelvis.

1. Describe four abnormalities you may see in the X-ray.
2. What pharmacological agents would you begin with? If these don't work, what is your next plan of action?
3. Name three non-pharmacological management options for OA.
4. She returns to your clinic some months later complaining that the medications are not working. What are the indications for surgical intervention and what procedure should be performed?

Answers to self-assessment questions are to be found on the Resources tab at www.scionpublishing.com/Rheum2.

2.3 Septic arthritis

Septic arthritis is the **acute infection** (usually **bacterial**) of a **native** or **prosthetic joint**. Since septic arthritis can lead to **rapid joint destruction**, immediate accurate diagnosis and treatment are essential. Any joint can be affected, particularly the **lower limb joints**, most commonly the **hip** and **knee**. The presentation is typically mono- / oligo-arthritis (bacterial causes) but can be polyarthritis (viral causes).

Pathophysiology

- Septic arthritis usually occurs due to the spread of bacteria from another site to the joint:
  - The most common route of spread is **haematogenous** (**respiratory** or **urinary tract infection**). Highly vascularized joints lack a limiting basement membrane, making them more vulnerable.
  - Other routes include **local tissue infection** (**cellulitis** and **osteomyelitis**), **penetrating trauma** and **inoculation** (skin opportunistic pathogens may spread when there is a break in the skin).
- Release of **cytokines by osteoclasts and synovial macrophages** leads to hydrolysis of **proteoglycans** and **collagen**. **Cartilage destruction** and eventual **bone loss** (if left untreated) begin within 48 hours, and are caused by direct invasion by the causative agent resulting in increased intra-articular pressure.
- **Bacteria** are the most common causative pathogens (*Fig. 2.3.1*). **Viruses** and **fungi** rarely cause septic arthritis.

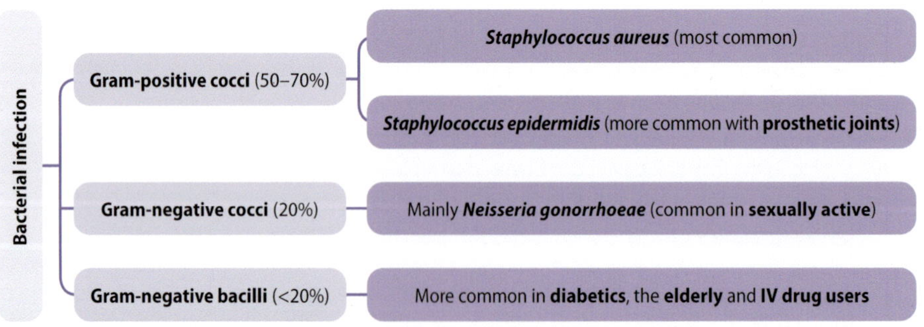

Fig. 2.3.1: Causative bacteria of septic arthritis.

Epidemiology and risk factors

- The estimated incidence of septic arthritis in the UK is 7.8 cases per 100 000 of the population (2016) (https://doi.org/10.1093/rheumatology/kew323).

Table 2.3.1: Risk factors for septic arthritis

Prosthetic joint	• Incidence is 10 × higher. Early infection is most likely due to *Staphylococcus aureus*, whereas delayed infection is due to coagulase-negative staphylococcus and Gram-negative aerobes.
Rheumatoid arthritis	• Incidence is 4 × higher.
Diabetes mellitus	• Diabetic patients have increased risk of infection; this can often be linked to foot ulcers.
Low socioeconomic status	• Poverty and malnutrition, and those abusing alcohol and drugs.
Age	• Extremes of age (<15 and >80).
Intravenous drug use	• Transfer of pathogenic organisms via haematogenous spread; joints of the spine are more often affected.
Osteomyelitis	• Osteomyelitis from penetrating injuries can spread to joint.
Intra-articular injection / aspiration	• Transfer of pathogenic skin organisms directly into joint.

Clinical features

Rapid diagnosis: Septic arthritis in children (Kocher criteria for a child with a painful hip)

- Non-weight-bearing on affected side
- Raised ESR and/or CRP
- Fever
- Raised WCC

Probability that child has septic arthritis: 4/4 = 99%, 3/4 = 93%, 2/4 = 40%, 1/4 = 3%

- Usually **one joint** is affected (approx. 90% of the time). Less commonly two or more joints may be affected at the same time due to the spread of bacteria.
- The **knee** is the most common site of infection (**>50%**), followed by the **hip** (more common in **children**), then the **shoulder**, **wrist**, **elbow** and **ankle**. Other joints are rarely affected, but hand and foot may be infected after bacterial infection following piercing trauma.

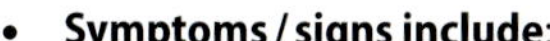

- **Symptoms / signs include**:

  - **Extremely painful, red (erythema), swollen joint (acute).**
  - **Muscle spasm** resulting in **joint immobility**.
  - **Systemic features** – tachycardia, fever, rash, malaise, anorexia.
  - **Loosening of the implant** (chronic infection in prosthetic joint).
  - **Reduced passive joint mobility**.
- The clinical picture may be partially masked in the **elderly**, **immunocompromised**, those with **RA** and **IV drug users**.

Diagnosis and investigations

Hx

- **Presenting complaint**: extreme pain, overlying skin is red, swollen joint and fever (60%). In most cases of septic arthritis there is a rapid onset of symptoms (<2 weeks) and only one joint is affected.
- **Past medical history**: e.g. diabetes, RA and other risk factors (*Table 2.3.1*).
- **Social history**: low socioeconomic status and IV drug use.
- **Sexual history**: gonorrhoeal infection.

Ex

- **Look** → signs of erythema, swelling and obvious effusion.
- **Feel** → tenderness, warmth and effusion.
- **Move** → marked limitation of movements and inability to bear weight.
- Presence of **systemic features** (fever, malaise, rash and tachycardia).

Ix

- **Aspiration of the joint (image-guided if available)**: to obtain a sample of synovial fluid. Synovial fluid is sent for immediate Gram stain, WCC, culture and polarized light microscopy (to rule out gout / CPPD). May show presence of microorganisms; WCC is often raised. Subsequent culture reveals organism type and sensitivities to antibiotic therapy.
- **Blood culture**: presence of microorganisms; reveals organism type and sensitivities to antibiotic therapy.
- **Blood test**: ↑ESR, WCC and CRP. Electrolyte and liver function tests can be performed to indicate whether there is systemic sepsis.
- **X-ray**: usually normal but may reveal any underlying joint disease at presentation, e.g. RA. May show effusion and narrowing of joint space due to cartilage destruction.
- **Ultrasound**: may show presence of synovial thickening or effusion to guide aspiration.
- **CT with contrast and MRI**: useful for determining extent of infection.
- Other investigations to find the source of infection may be useful, such as **MSU or urethral swabs**.

DDx

- Gout
- Pseudogout
- Acute exacerbation of OA
- Bursitis
- Flare-up of RA
- Transient non-specific synovitis (hip)
- Reactive arthritis
- Haemarthrosis

Management

Antibiotics

- **Empirical antibiotics** (initially **IV**) whilst waiting for synovial fluid joint analysis (refer to local guidelines and consult microbiologist).
- The choice of empirical therapy depends on the most likely causative organism:
  - **Flucloxacillin** (0.5–1 g/6 hours IV for 4–6 weeks) for ***Staphylococcus aureus*** and **vancomycin** for **MRSA**.
  - If **penicillin-allergic** then **IV vancomycin** should be given (dose variable adjusted to trough level (15–20 mg/L)).
  - **Cefotaxime** (1 g every 12 hours IV for 4–6 weeks) for **gonococcal** or **Gram-negative bacteria**.
- Other antibiotics may be indicated and added, depending on the results of culture and sensitivity testing.
- Antibiotic therapy (initially IV then later oral) should be continued for at least **1 week and longer where clinically indicated**.

Non-pharmacological management

- **Orthopaedic review** for the consideration of **arthrocentesis**, **lavage** and **debridement**, particularly if **prosthetic joint** is affected.
- **Joint immobilization** followed by **physiotherapy**.
- **Regular review** and **examination** of the affected joint as well as follow-up blood tests for inflammatory markers.

Self-assessment

A 9 year old boy presents with an acute red, swollen hip and is unable to walk. You suspect that he has septic arthritis.

1. What findings would you expect on examination?
2. What is the most common route of spread in septic arthritis?
3. Name three risk factors of septic arthritis.
4. An aspiration of the joint is performed to obtain a sample of synovial fluid. What tests should be performed on the sample?
5. What is the most likely causative organism for sepsis in this case?
6. What suitable empirical antibiotic would you prescribe?

Answers to self-assessment questions are to be found on the Resources tab at www.scionpublishing.com/Rheum2.

Introduction to spondyloarthropathies

- Spondyloarthropathies are a group of inflammatory arthropathies which include the following conditions ('**PEAR**'):
  - **Psoriatic arthritis** (*Sec. 2.4*)
  - **Enteropathic spondyloarthropathies** – associated with inflammatory bowel disease and GI bypass surgery (this condition is not discussed any further in this book)
  - **Ankylosing spondylitis** (*Sec. 2.5*)
  - **Reactive arthritis** (*Sec. 2.6*)
- The spondyloarthropathies frequently overlap and have several clinical features in common:
  - **Rheumatoid factor negative** (seronegative)
  - **HLA-B27 association** – HLA-B27-positive individuals have a 20-fold increased risk of developing a spondyloarthropathy
  - **Axial arthritis** – arthritis of the spine and sacroiliac joints
  - **Asymmetrical large joint oligoarthritis** (<5 joints) or **monoarthritis**
  - **Enthesitis** – inflammation of the site of tendon or ligament insertion e.g. plantar fasciitis and Achilles tendinitis
  - **Dactylitis** ('sausage digit') – inflammation of the entire digit as a result of soft tissue oedema, and tenosynovial and joint inflammation
  - **Extra-articular manifestations** – these differ from RA, e.g. inflammatory bowel disease (IBD) and iritis

The European Spondyloarthropathy Study Group criteria for spondyloarthropathy 1991

Inflammatory spinal pain, or **synovitis** (asymmetric, predominantly in the lower extremities) and one or more of the following:

- **Family history**: first-degree or second-degree relative with **ankylosing spondylitis**, **psoriasis**, **acute iritis**, **reactive arthritis** or **IBD**
- Past or present **psoriasis**
- Past or present **IBD**
- Past or present pain alternating between the two buttocks
- Past or present spontaneous **enthesitis** on examination
- Episode of diarrhoea occurring within one month before onset of arthritis
- **Non-gonococcal urethritis** or **cervicitis** occurring within one month before onset of arthritis
- **Sacroiliitis** (meeting the criteria shown in *Fig. 2.5.2*)

2.4 Psoriatic arthritis

Psoriatic arthritis (PsA) is a **chronic inflammatory arthritis** and the most common type of **seronegative oligoarthritis**. PsA is unique compared to other **seronegative spondyloarthritides** in that the **small joints** of the **hand** are commonly affected. A variety of joint patterns are recognized in PsA, although these may overlap. It affects up to 25% of people with psoriasis; the risk correlates to the severity of psoriasis.

Pathophysiology

- The pathogenesis of PsA remains poorly understood.
- Like other autoimmune joint diseases, **genetically susceptible individuals** are exposed to an **environmental trigger** (**bacteria**, **stress**, or **entheseal-related peptide**) which may then activate the immune system.
- This results in **T-cell infiltration** and **chemokine / cytokine** release, and hyperplasia of the synovium.
- The process is amplified by **angiogenesis**, **cellular infiltration (B cells and macrophages), and fibrosis** of involved tissues.
- **Human leucocyte antigen (HLA)** and other genes may determine the exact pattern of tissue involvement.
- **Plasmacytoid cells may play a key role in the pathogenesis of PsA**.
- **Osteoclast activity** is also increased in PsA, leading to **bone remodelling**.

Epidemiology and risk factors

- The prevalence of PsA in the UK is approximately 0.3%.
- Incidence has been observed in studies to be around 16 per 100 000 people in the UK.
- Men and women are equally affected.

Table 2.4.1: Risk factors for PsA

Psoriasis	**Strongest risk factor**. Skin psoriasis may occur **before** (**70%**), **after** (**15%**), or at **same time as** (**15%**) joint symptoms.
Hereditary	Approx. **30%** of individuals with psoriasis or PsA have first-degree relatives with psoriasis or PsA. There is an association between **HLA-B27** and PsA.
Joint or tendon trauma	A small number of PsA patients may recall trauma prior to the onset of their arthritis.
HIV	The prevalence of PsA is higher in patients with HIV compared to the general population.
Age	More common in individuals aged **30–55** but can occur at any age.
Ethnicity	PsA is more common in **Caucasians** than Africans or Asians.

Clinical features

- A variety of PsA patterns of joint involvement are recognized (*Table 2.4.2*).

Table 2.4.2: Patterns of PsA – 'DR SAM'

DIP joint disease (5–10%)	Predominantly **DIP** involvement (*Fig. 2.4.1*). Affects **men** more and is strongly associated with **onycholysis**.
Rheumatoid pattern (25%)	Presents very similarly to RA – **symmetrical small joint arthritis** particularly affecting **MCP**, **wrist** and **PIP joints**. Distinguishing features are **lack of nodules** and **negative** for **RF**.
Spondyloarthritis (20%)	May present with isolated **sacroiliitis**, **typical** or **atypical AS**.
Asymmetrical oligoarthritis (50%)	**Large joint inflammatory arthritis** often with **ankle**, **knee**, **wrist** or **shoulder** involvement.
Mutilans arthritis (1–5%)	Most **rare** but **severe** form. **Osteolysis** results in **destruction** of the **small joints** of the **digits** with **shortening** (*Fig. 2.4.2*).

- **General symptoms and signs**:
  - **Joint pain** and **stiffness** – inflammatory joint pain is characterized by prolonged morning stiffness (>30 mins), improvement with use, and recurrence with prolonged rest.
  - **Dactylitis** or '**sausage digits**' (*Fig. 2.4.3*).
  - **Enthesitis** – pain, stiffness and tenderness of insertions into bone e.g. the Achilles tendon (*Fig. 2.4.4*).
  - Extra-articular features – **psoriatic skin rash** (*Fig. 2.4.5*), **nail changes** (pitting, onycholysis and hyperkeratosis) and **uveitis**.
- **The Psoriasis Epidemiological Screening Tool** (PEST) can be used to assess for PsA in patients with psoriasis. It consists of questions relating to joint pain, swelling, fingernail pitting and heel pain.

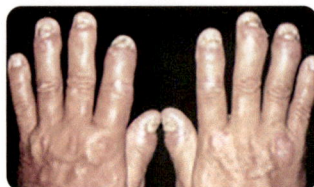

Fig. 2.4.1: DIP involvement in PsA – highly characteristic.

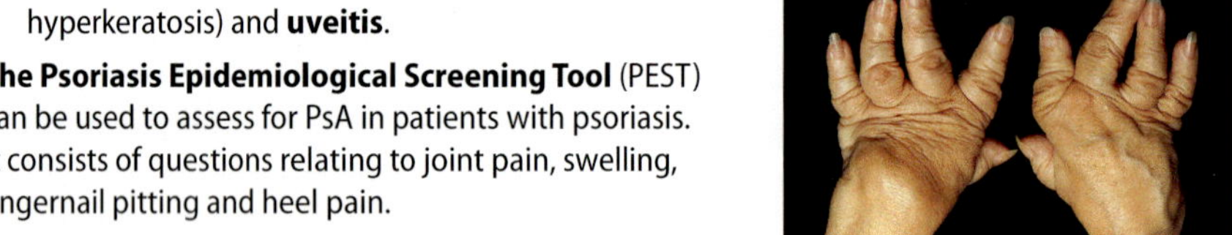

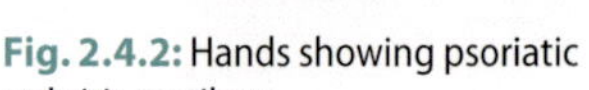

Fig. 2.4.2: Hands showing psoriatic arthritis mutilans.

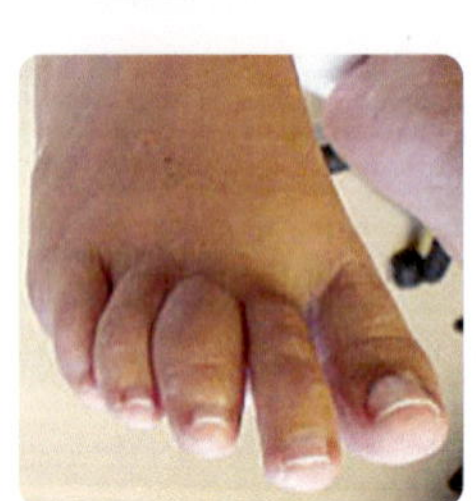

Fig. 2.4.3: 'Sausage toes'.

Rapid diagnosis: Classification Criteria for Psoriatic Arthritis (CASPAR) 2006

Established inflammatory articular disease and ≥3 points is diagnostic of PsA:

A. **Current psoriasis** = 2 points
B. **History of psoriasis** (in the absence of A) = 1
C. **Family history of psoriasis** (in the absence of A or B) = 1
D. **Dactylitis** = 1
E. **Juxta-articular new bone formation** = 1
F. **RF negative** = 1
G. **Nail dystrophy** = 1

Diagnosis and investigations

Hx

- **Clinical presentation** (*see above*).
- **Family history** – psoriasis or psoriatic arthritis.
- **Past medical history** – psoriasis, history of scalp or nail problems, joint or tendon trauma and HIV.

Ex

- Recognition of the pattern of joint involvement is essential to the diagnosis of PsA (*Table 2.4.2*).
- **Swelling and tenderness** of individual joints (synovitis) during inspection and palpation.
- **'Sausage digits'**.
- **Skin**, **scalp** and **nail** involvement – patients may not know they have psoriasis!
- **Pain at site of tendon attachment** – commonly affected sites include **Achilles tendon**, **plantar fascia**, and **epicondyles**.
- **Spinal stiffness** with low back pain due to **sacroiliitis** (uncommon).

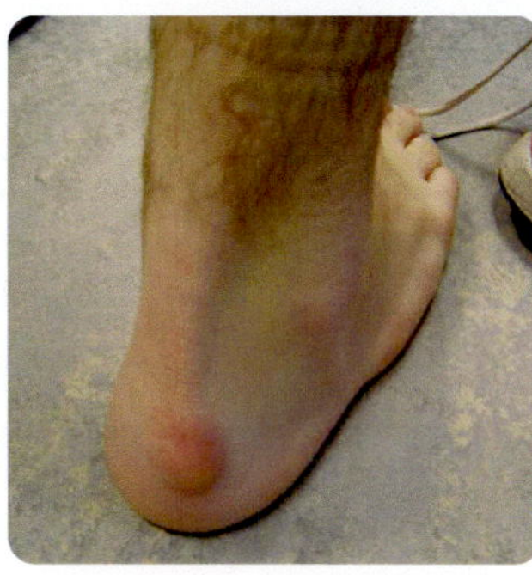

Fig. 2.4.4: Achilles tendon bursitis.

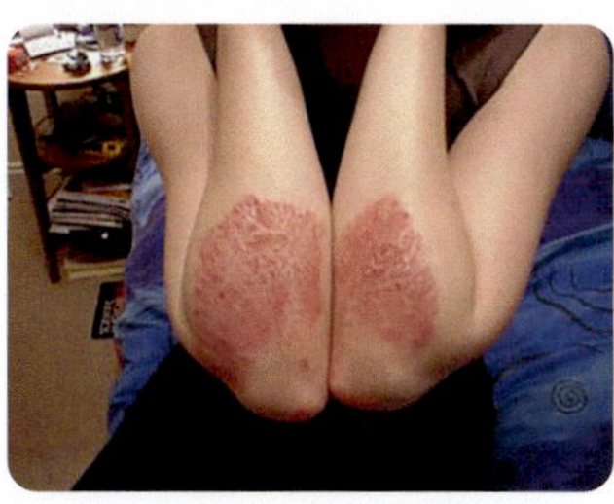

Fig. 2.4.5: Psoriatic skin rash.

Ix

1. **X-rays**:
   - Soft tissue swelling may be the only radiographical finding seen in early disease.
   - Erosion in the DIP joint and periarticular new-bone formation; osteolysis and 'pencil-in-cup' deformity in advanced disease (*Fig. 2.4.6*).
2. **Blood tests**:
   - Normal or raised ESR and CRP (in active disease).
   - Immunology – RF, anti-CCP and antinuclear antibodies (ANA) negative.

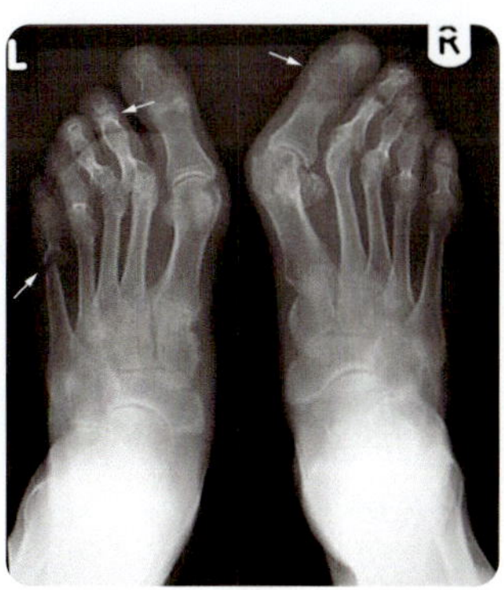

Fig. 2.4.6: Arrows show 'pencil-in-cup' deformity caused by underlying osteolysis.

DDx

- RA (symmetrical pattern)
- Erosive OA
- Gout (monoarthritic, large joint, especially knee)
- Reactive arthritis
- Sarcoid dactylitis

Management

Treatment depends upon PsA severity, impact on patient's life, risk factors. **Mild disease** may only involve **oligoarthritis** or have **limited psoriasis. Severe disease** may be **erosive**, **cause major impairment to quality of life, be function-limiting**, or cause **joint deformities**. Patients suspected of having PsA should be referred to a rheumatologist for confirmation of diagnosis and initiating management.

Table 2.4.3: Management of PsA

NSAIDs	First-line for **pain relief** and **soft tissue inflammation**.
cDMARDs	• First-line for those with **progressive peripheral joint disease** who require more aggressive treatment. • **Methotrexate** is usually the first-line DMARD. • Alternative DMARDs include **ciclosporin**, **sulfasalazine** and **leflunomide**. • The combination of methotrexate and ciclosporin is particularly effective. • An initial trial of a DMARD for PsA is **3 months**. • DMARDs require monitoring and possibly lifestyle advice to reduce modifiable risk factors.
Intra-articular corticosteroid injections	• May be indicated if NSAIDs alone are not sufficient for symptomatic relief. • Corticosteroid injection is given once and then reassessed.
Anti-TNF-α therapy	• Highly effective for **severe skin** and **joint disease**. • Reduces radiographic progression of PsA. • There is no preferred TNF-α inhibitor – **etanercept**, **adalimumab**, **infliximab** or **golimumab** can be used. • Apremilast is a selective inhibitor of phosphodiesterase 4 (PDE4) and inhibits spontaneous production of TNF-α.
Anti-IL17 or 23/12 agents (bDMARD)	• Similar results to anti-TNF; however, there may be a slightly improved skin response. • Secukinumab (targets IL-17), ustekinumab (targets IL-12 and IL-23).
JAK inhibitor	• Tofacitinib selectively inhibits JAK1 and JAK3. • Can be considered after cDMARD if bDMARD is ineffective or unable to be used. • Reduces radiographic progression of PsA. • A risk assessment should be completed before use.
Physiotherapy	Helps improve range of motion and pain, as well as muscle strengthening of joints with associated periarticular muscle atrophy.
Occupational therapy	• Workplace adaptations. • Equipment provision to help with daily activities.

Self-assessment

A 52 year old male with a past medical history of psoriasis complains of symmetrical pain and swelling in both of his hands. You suspect psoriatic arthritis.

1. Apart from psoriatic skin rash, name two other extra-articular features of psoriatic arthritis.
2. What clinical features distinguish rheumatoid arthritis from psoriatic arthritis?
3. What blood tests help to distinguish between rheumatoid arthritis and psoriatic arthritis?
4. An X-ray is later performed. What abnormalities might you see?
5. Name two analgesic options for patients with psoriatic arthritis, and two classes of disease-modifying drugs.
6. Name the first-line pharmacological agent to prevent disease progression and its side-effects.

Answers to self-assessment questions are to be found on the Resources tab at www.scionpublishing.com/Rheum2.

2.5 Ankylosing spondylitis

Ankylosing spondylitis (AS) is one of the more severe **seronegative axial spondyloarthropathies (AxSpA)**. AxSpA may have radiographic changes (r-AxSpA) or characteristic clinical features without radiographic changes (nr-AxSpA). AS is a **chronic inflammatory** disorder of the **sacroiliac joints** and **spine** with **significant radiographic change**.

Other clinical features include **peripheral arthritis**, **enthesitis** and **extra-articular organ** involvement.

Pathophysiology

Fig. 2.5.1: **(a)** Normal spine, **(b)** early AS, **(c)** advanced AS.

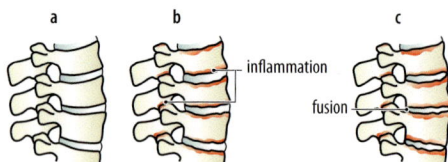

- Both **genetic** and **environmental** factors interplay in the pathogenesis of AS. In particular, **TNF** and **IL-17/23** are indicated to play an important role in pathogenesis through treatment response.
- **HLA-B27** is the most common predisposing gene in AS and has a **direct role** in progression; however, this is poorly understood. In ~90% of patients there is subclinical intestinal inflammation, which is related to HLA-B27. This leads to the overproduction of interleukins and may allow more systemic exposure to pathogens which may affect AS.
- The disease is first characterized by **inflammation** of the **sacroiliac (SI) joints** and more generally follows an **autoinflammatory** disease progression.
- **T cells** play a key role in AS and many infiltrate the synovium of the SI joints (along with elevated levels of **TNF**). **γδ T cells** (expressing **IL-17/23 receptors)** are also present at high levels, particularly in the spinal enthesis.
- SI joint involvement is followed by involvement of several structures including the **intervertebral discs**, **zygapophyseal**, **costovertebral** and the **costotransverse joints**, as well as the **paravertebral ligaments**.
- Early lesions include **subchondral granulation tissue** which erodes the joint and is replaced gradually by **fibrocartilage** and then ossification. This occurs in **ligamentous** and **capsular** attachment sites to bone (**enthesitis**). The threshold for enthesitis to occur is lowered in patients with AS.
- In the later stage, the outer layer of the **annulus fibrosis** starts to **calcify**, creating a bony bridge between the **vertebral bodies (syndesmophytes)**.
- These may then fuse with the vertebral body above, causing **ankylosis** ('**bamboo spine**') (*Fig. 2.5.3*).

Epidemiology and risk factors

- AS is one of the more common seronegative AxSpA, with a prevalence of 150 per 100 000 in the UK.
- A number of patients with mild symptoms remain undiagnosed.

Table 2.5.1: Risk factors for ankylosing spondylitis	
Genetics	• 90% of AS patients carry the **HLA-B27 gene**.
Gender	• Affects men more than women **(2:1)**.
Age	• Peaks at ages **20–30** and typically occurs <45.
Family	• First-degree relative correlates to a **5.6–16× increase in risk**.

Clinical features

- **Dull back pain** (radiating from the SI joints to the hips / buttocks) and **stiffness** >3 months. These symptoms are worse at night and in the early morning, and are relieved by exercise and worsened by rest.
- **Reduced motion** in the **lumbar spine**, and **cervical spine movements** can be globally reduced.
- Loss of **lumbar lordosis**.
- **Reduced chest expansion** due to progressive loss of spinal movements.
- **Thoracic kyphosis** and **neck hyperextension** ('**question mark posture**') – uncommon and occurs with progressive disease.
- **Peripheral synovitis** (approx. 30%). Typically, asymmetrical oligoarthritis, most commonly affecting the hip and knee.
- **Extra-articular features** (*Box 2.5.1*).

Box 2.5.1: Extra-articular features of AS ('The A factor')

- Atlanto-axial subluxation
- Anterior uveitis (25.8%)
- Apical lung fibrosis
- Aortic incompetence
- AV (atrioventricular) node block
- Achilles tendinitis
- Amyloidosis (a rare and late complication)

Other common features include **psoriasis** (9.3%) and **IBD** (6.8%).

OSCE tips: Schober's test

- The modified Schober's test examines flexion of the spine.
- An inferior mark at the level of **posterior superior iliac spines** is drawn and a **10 cm** segment above this point is marked on the patient's back.
- The increase in distance on maximal forward spinal flexion with **locked knees** is measured.
- The measured distance should increase from 10 cm to at least **13.5–15 cm** in healthy adults.

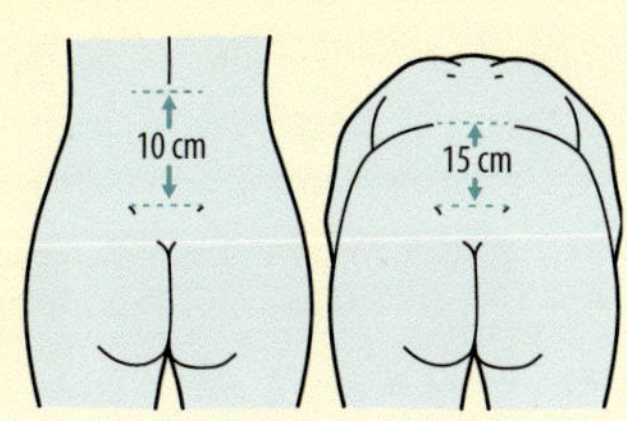

Diagnosis and investigations

- Based on the **modified New York (NY) criteria**, a definite diagnosis of AS requires the presence of radiological criteria and at least one clinical criterion (history and examination). Alternatively, HLA-B27 (+) and at least two of the ASAS (Assessment of SpondyloArthritis International Society) criteria (see the *Introduction to spondyloarthritis* section above) can also be used to diagnose AS.

Hx History of **back pain** and **stiffness** for longer than **3 months** which improves with exercise but is not relieved by rest.

Ex

NY

- **Limitation of motion** of the **lumbar spine** in both **sagittal** and **frontal planes** (see *OSCE tips*).
- **Limitation of chest expansion** to 1 inch or less.

ASAS

- See *Introduction to spondyloarthritis* section above.

Ix

- **X-ray** (modified NY radiological criterion): **sacroiliitis grade ≥2 bilaterally** or **grade 3** or **4 unilaterally** (see *Fig. 2.5.2* for sacroiliitis grading).
- Other radiographic features include:
  - **Early**: bone erosions, widening of the SI joints and vertebral bodies appear square with shiny corners (Romanus lesions).
  - **Later**: ossification of longitudinal ligaments of the spine (syndesmophytes) giving it a 'bamboo spine' appearance (*Fig. 2.5.3*).
- **MRI scanning**: although not included in the modified NY criteria, it is very useful for identifying early sacroiliitis and early inflammatory changes affecting the spine and therefore it can pick up AS at the early stages of the disease.
- **Blood tests**: FBC normal, ↑CRP and ESR (active disease), RF and ANA negative, HLA-B27 (this has little role in diagnosis, but may indicate a predisposition to AS in the appropriate clinical context).
- **Ultrasound scanning**: can help in diagnosing enthesitis.

DDx

- Mechanical back pain
- Other seronegative AxSpAs
- Degenerative lumbar or cervical spondylosis
- Trauma
- Infection
- Neoplasm

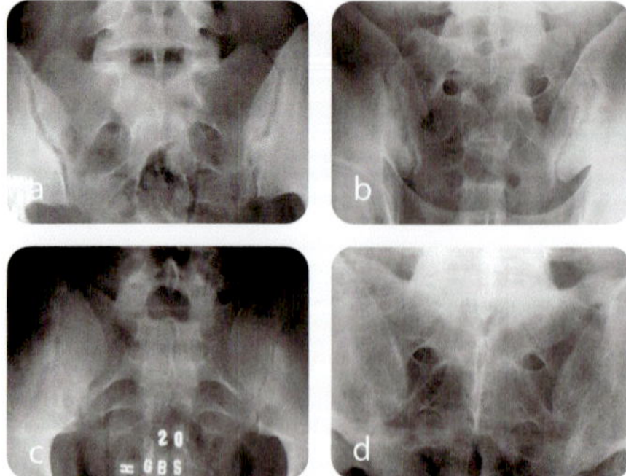

Fig. 2.5.2: Grading of sacroiliitis: **(a)** grade 0, normal; **(b)** grade I–II, mild sclerosis; **(c)** grade III, widening of joint space; **(d)** grade IV, bilateral ankylosis.

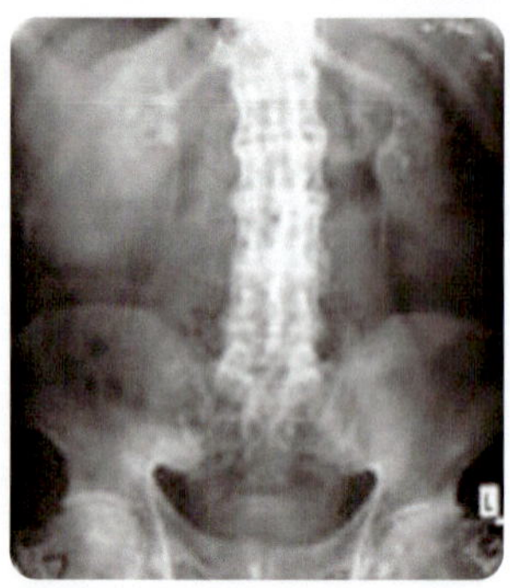

Fig. 2.5.3: X-ray of 'bamboo spine' in AS.

Management

- Early diagnosis and patient education are essential for effective AS management (*Table 2.5.2*).
- The goal of treatment is to maximize health-related quality of life over the long term.

Table 2.5.2: Management of AS based on Assessment of SpondyloArthritis International Society (ASAS) / European Alliance of Associations for Rheumatology (EULAR) recommendations

Exercise, physiotherapy, and education	Intense exercises or activities such as badminton and swimming to strengthen muscle and provide better stability. The National Axial Spondyloarthritis Society (NASS) can be signposted for patient information. Disease activity monitoring is essential.
NSAIDs	First-line therapy for AS patients with pain and stiffness. Relieves symptoms and may slow radiographic progression. Examples – ibuprofen and naproxen.
Other analgesics	Offered when NSAIDs are insufficient or contraindicated. Examples – codeine and paracetamol.
Local corticosteroids	Temporarily relieve pain that does not respond well to NSAIDs if peripheral symptoms are also present.
Anti-TNF-α therapy	Given to patients with persistently high disease activity or if NSAIDs fail. Examples – adalimumab, etanercept and golimumab.
IL-17i	Given to patients with persistently high disease activity or if NSAIDs fail. Preferred over TNF inhibitor if psoriasis is present.
JAKi	Typically given after other bDMARDs have been trialled without success.
Surgery	Hip replacements are offered to patients with advanced hip involvement who suffer from refractory pain and disability. Spinal deformity correction surgery can also be considered if quality of life is being affected. Surgery should also be considered for cauda equina and for spinal fractures.

- A tool called the **Bath Ankylosing Spondylitis Disease Activity Index (BASDAI)** has been formulated for measuring the disease activity of AS by asking 6 questions related to 5 major symptoms of AS: **fatigue**, **spinal pain**, **arthralgia**, **enthesitis** and **morning stiffness**.
- **The Ankylosing Spondylitis Disease Activity Score with CRP (ASDAS–CRP)** is another alternative. This consists of 5 questions relating to **back pain, morning stiffness, patient global assessment, peripheral pain**, and **CRP/ESR** level.

Self-assessment

A 22 year old male presents with low back pain and stiffness that has persisted for more than 3 months. His back symptoms are worse when he awakes in the morning, and the stiffness lasts more than 1 hour. There is no history of obvious injury.

1. What condition do you think this man has and why?
2. What special test would you perform on clinical examination? Describe how this is performed.
3. Which gene is strongly linked to the likely cause of his presentation?
4. What abnormalities might you see if an X-ray is performed on this man's lower back?
5. Outline a management plan for this patient.

Answers to self-assessment questions are to be found on the Resources tab at www.scionpublishing.com/Rheum2.

2.6 Reactive arthritis

Reactive arthritis (ReA) is an **acute aseptic arthritis** that develops in response to an extra-articular infection, typically originating from the **gastrointestinal (GI)** or **genitourinary (GU) tract**. It is a **seronegative spondyloarthropathy** classically presenting with **asymmetrical oligoarthritis**, usually in the **lower limbs**.

Pathophysiology

- Reactive arthritis is thought to be caused by an **infectious trigger**, usually a **bacterial GI** or **GU infection** (*Fig. 2.6.1*) in **genetically susceptible individuals**. These bacterial products can infiltrate the synovium.
- This leads to **immune activation** and **cross-reactivity** with **self-antigens** causing **acute inflammation** in the affected joint and other tissues approximately **2–6 weeks** after the initial infection. The length of time which bacterial components remain in the synovium is a factor in whether ReA progresses into chronic arthritis.

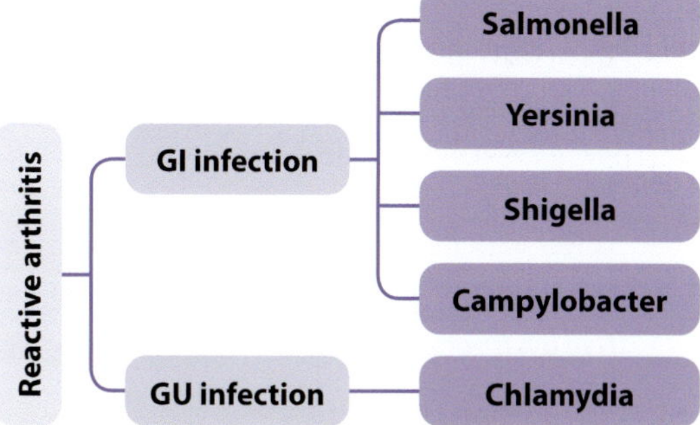

Fig. 2.6.1: The key GI and GU bacteria implicated in reactive arthritis.

- As well as inflammation of joints, inflammation of the **entheses**, **axial skeleton**, **skin**, **mucous membranes**, **GI tract** and **eyes** may also occur.
- **HLA-B27** is positive in most patients, and it is not only a strong risk factor of reactive arthritis, but it may also predict the severity and chronicity of the disease. HLA-B27 (+), which prolongs the intracellular lifespan of some bacteria, may increase the risk of induced T lymphocytes invading joints.

Epidemiology and risk factors

- The estimated incidence of reactive arthritis in the UK is approximately 30–40 cases per 100 000 of the population.
- The incidence of ReA for Chlamydia- and enterobacteria-induced arthritis is 4.6 and 5 per 100 000 per year, respectively.

Table 2.6.1: Risk factors for reactive arthritis

GI / GU infection	Reactive arthritis occurs after exposure to certain GI or GU infections.
Gender	There is a **9:1 male:female** incidence ratio of **Chlamydia-induced reactive arthritis** and **1:1** for **post-dysentery reactive arthritis**.
HLA-B27	HLA-B27 is positive in approximately 50% of reactive arthritis patients overall. This is significantly higher in ReA following *Shigella*, *Yersinia* or *Chlamydia* (60–85%) and lower following *Salmonella* and *Campylobacter*.
Age	Most patients with reactive arthritis are **aged 20–40**.
Ethnicity	Reactive arthritis is more common in **Caucasians**; however, it is often the first sign of HIV infection in Africans and does not have an association with HLA-B27.

Clinical features

- **Arthritis** – acute, asymmetrical large joint arthritis (often lower limbs), occurring 2–6 weeks after the initial infection (most often acute, and may be accompanied by malaise, fatigue and fever).
- Other features:
  - **Enthesitis** – plantar fasciitis and Achilles tendinitis.
  - **Conjunctivitis** (usually bilateral and painful) and **anterior uveitis** (usually unilateral).
  - **Dactylitis** – may occur at one or more toes.
  - **Urethritis** (dysuria, frequency and discharge) and **circinate balanitis** (ulcers and vesicles surrounding the glans penis).
  - **Prostatitis or cervicitis**.
  - **Lower back pain** due to sacroiliitis and spondylitis. This is relatively common following ReA.
  - **Mouth ulcers**.
  - **Nail dystrophy** and **keratoderma blennorrhagica** (*Fig. 2.6.2*).
  - **Reiter's syndrome** – triad of **reactive arthritis**, **conjunctivitis** and **urethritis**. Although rare, it follows a GU or GI infection. It can be easily remembered using the mnemonic 'can't see, can't wee and can't bend your knee'!
  - **Rare cardiac complications include** aortitis (with or without aortic regurgitation) and conduction defects.

Diagnosis and investigations

Hx

- **Presenting complaints**: peripheral arthritis, axial arthritis (sacroiliitis), systemic features (fever, fatigue and weight loss) and enthesitis are all common.
- **History of GI or GU infection** prior to infection.
- **Family history** of reactive arthritis.
- Consider a **sexual health review**.

Ex

- **Examine the affected joint(s)**.
- **Eyes** – conjunctivitis and uveitis.
- **Mouth** – oral ulcers.
- **Lower back** – pain due to sacroiliitis.
- **Genitals** – urethritis and circinate balanitis.
- **Foot** – plantar fasciitis, Achilles tendinitis, keratoderma blennorrhagica, 'sausage toes' and nail dystrophy.
- **Systemic features** – malaise, fatigue and fever.

Working downwards anatomically

Ix

- **Blood tests**: raised CRP, ESR, leucocytosis and thrombocytosis (acute phase), ANA, RF and anti-CCP are negative, HLA-B27 positive in 50%.
- **X-ray**: normal in early stages. Marginal erosions, plantar spurs, sacroiliitis and asymmetrical syndesmophytes may occur in chronic cases.
- **Joint aspiration**: to rule out crystal or septic arthritis. Synovial fluid is usually sterile and cloudy with high WCC.
- **Stool, throat or urine culture**: identify causative organism.
- **Serology**: for Chlamydia.
- **MRI**: asymmetrical sacroiliitis and enthesitis (chronic stage).

DDx

- Other seronegative spondyloarthropathies
- Gonococcal arthritis
- Gout
- Inflammatory bowel disease
- RA
- Septic arthritis

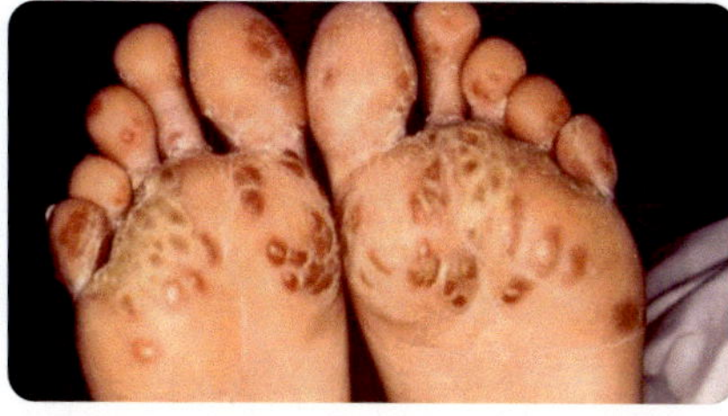

Fig. 2.6.2: Keratoderma blennorrhagica of the soles.

OSCE tips: Specific questions to ask someone with suspected reactive arthritis

- **Presenting complaint is usually asymmetrical joint pain**: Is it warm? Red? Sudden onset? Occurred after a bowel or urine infection? If so, how many days / weeks after?
- **Other complaints** (head to toe): Eye infection? Mouth ulcers? Back pain? Urine infection? Rash on penis? Pain or rash on soles of feet? Swollen toes? Fatigue? Fever?
- **Past medical history**: Recent stomach bug or urine infection?
- **Family history**: Has anyone in your family suffered from anything similar?
- **Sexual history**: Unprotected sex? New partner?

Management

- Reactive arthritis usually lasts between 3 months and 1 year.

Table 2.6.2: Management of reactive arthritis

Non-pharmacological	**Rest** and **splint** affected joint (acutely). Consider **physiotherapy**.
NSAIDs	For **pain relief** and **soft tissue inflammation**.
Corticosteroids	**Intra-articular**, for instance **sacroiliac joints** can be injected. A short course of **oral corticosteroids** can be considered for patients who are unresponsive to NSAIDs or who develop adverse effects. **Topical corticosteroids** can be used to treat skin involvement.
cDMARDs	Particularly **methotrexate** and **sulfasalazine** have been shown to be beneficial for some patients; indicated for **persistent** or **refractory disease**.
Antibiotics	**Tetracyclines** may be useful for **urethritis** caused by **Chlamydia**. Antibiotics are generally not indicated for uncomplicated GI infections.
Anti-TNF-α therapy	In more aggressive cases, or when reactive arthritis evolves towards AxSpA (chronic), anti-TNF-α therapy may represent an effective choice.

Self-assessment

A 21 year old male presents with a 2 week history of an acute painful, hot, and swollen left knee, and low back pain with bilateral buttock pain. Further review of symptoms indicates the patient was treated for a Chlamydia infection after he developed dysuria approximately 2 months ago. You suspect reactive arthritis.

1. What risk factors predispose this patient to reactive arthritis?
2. On examination, why would you look at the soles of the feet?
3. What is the name of the reactive arthritis manifestation shown in *Fig. 2.6.3*?
4. What blood tests would you perform and what do you expect to find?
5. How would you manage this patient acutely?

Answers to self-assessment questions are to be found on the Resources tab at www.scionpublishing.com/Rheum2.

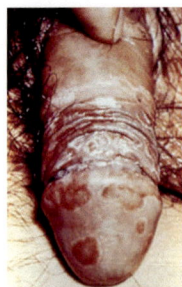

Fig. 2.6.3: Reactive arthritis manifestation.

2.7 Gout

Gout is an episodic **inflammatory arthritis** which progresses from asymptomatic **hyperuricaemia** (elevated circulating **uric acid levels**). It is caused by deposition of **urate crystals** in the **synovial fluid** of **joints**, **bone** and other tissues.

Pathophysiology

- There is an association between gouty arthropathy and **hyperuricaemia** which is **often asymptomatic** for up to **20 years** before the initial attack (*Fig. 2.7.1*).

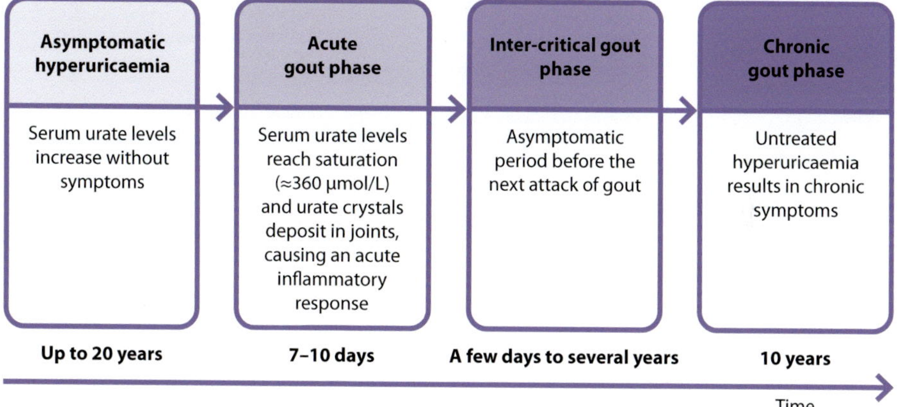

Asymptomatic hyperuricaemia
Serum urate levels increase without symptoms
Acute gout phase
Serum urate levels reach saturation (≈360 µmol/L) and urate crystals deposit in joints, causing an acute inflammatory response
Inter-critical gout phase
Asymptomatic period before the next attack of gout
Chronic gout phase
Untreated hyperuricaemia results in chronic symptoms
Up to 20 years
7–10 days
A few days to several years
10 years
Time

Fig. 2.7.1: Timescale of gout development.

- The build-up of **urate crystal** (a purine product) can be caused by **impaired renal excretion**, **overproduction of uric acid** and/or by **overconsumption of purine-rich foods** that are metabolized to **urate**.
- This can progress to **gouty arthritis**, where there is long-term synovitis and bone deformities due to erosion. **Monosodium urate (MSU) crystals** are broken down by leucocytes resulting in the release of enzymes, inflammatory mediators, and further leucocyte recruitment causing persistent synovitis.

Epidemiology and risk factors

- The **prevalence** of gout in the **UK** is approximately **2.5%** and is **increasing** (more common in countries such as the USA) because of obesity and dietary factors.
- The incidence of gout in the UK is approximately 4.4 in men and 1.3 in women per 1000 person years.

Table 2.7.1: Risk factors for gout	
Hyperuricaemia	• The **most important risk factor** for gout (however, a high level does not confirm gout).
Male sex	• Approximately **4.3:1** male:female ratio. Females tend to present post-menopause.
Diet	• **Meat** (especially red meat) and **seafood** (especially shellfish).
Alcohol	• Alcohol is metabolized to **ketones** that compete with urate for renal excretion; alcohol also ↑ risk of gout via **dehydration**.
Drugs	• **Diuretics** (thiazide and loop), **aspirin**, **ciclosporin** and **laxatives**.
Chronic renal failure	• Inability to excrete urate.
Other risk factors	• **Obesity**, **hypertension**, **family history**, **age**, **coronary heart disease** and **diabetes mellitus**.

Clinical features

Most commonly affects the **first metatarso-phalangeal joint (MTP)** – gout here is also known as **podagra** (occurs in 70–90% of cases) (*Fig. 2.7.2a*). Other common sites include **small joints** of the **foot (mid-tarsal)** and **hand**, **the ankle**, **knee** and **elbow**.

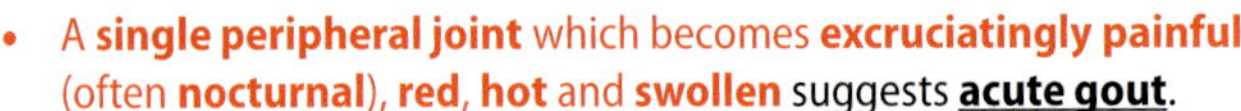

- A **single peripheral joint** which becomes **excruciatingly painful** (often **nocturnal**), **red**, **hot** and **swollen** suggests **acute gout**.
- **Polyarthritis**, **tophi** (nodular subcutaneous deposition of uric acid crystals, see *Fig. 2.7.2b* and *c*), **fever and malaise** (uncommon) suggest **chronic gout** (**uric acid kidney stones** may also develop).

OSCE tips: Key questions to ask patients with suspected gout

- First time? Timing of onset and duration? Is it painful when socks are worn? Night attacks – painful with bed covers?
- Family history of gout / other arthritic conditions?
- Do you suffer from diabetes, hypertension or kidney problems? Do you take 'water pills'?
- Have you had any recent tests that included the injection of dye?
- Have you ever been told your serum urate levels are high?
- Diet habits and alcohol intake?

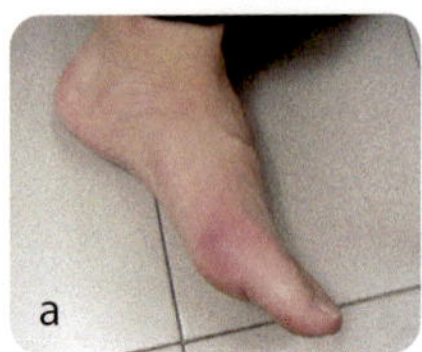

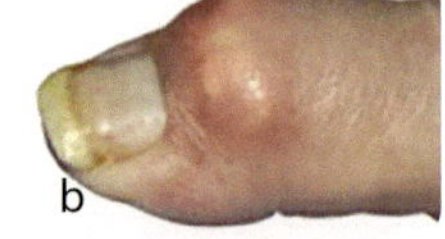

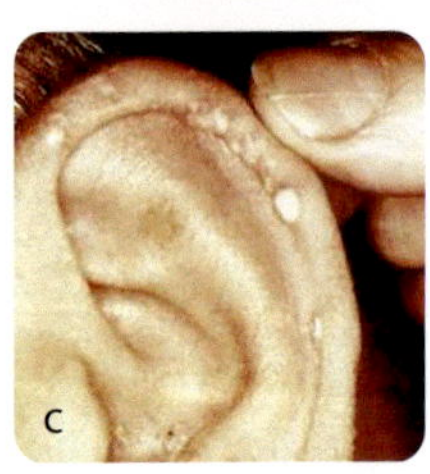

Fig. 2.7.2: (a) Gout of the big toe (podagra). Tophi affecting **(b)** DIP and **(c)** helix of the ear.

Diagnosis and investigations

Hx

- Typically, abrupt development of **severe joint pain** that reaches its maximum within **6–12 hours** and may undergo **remission** within **2 weeks (acute gout)**.
- **Risk factors** including age, family history, use of medication, diet and alcohol.

Ex

- **90%** of **gout attacks** are **monoarthritic**, and the majority occur in the **first MTP**.
- **Swelling, erythema, shiny surface and tenderness of the affected joint.**
- **Tophi** → **hallmark of chronic gout** (50% of people after 10 years of hyperuricaemia).

Ix

- **Joint aspiration (with US guidance where possible) and synovial fluid analysis** → definitive diagnosis demonstrated by the presence of negatively birefringent crystals under polarized light microscopy.
- **Serum urate measurement** → often elevated. Useful for monitoring the response to treatment.
- **USS** – can identify tophi or double contour sign on cartilage (highly specific for urate deposits and gout diagnosis).
- **Radiographs** – soft tissue swelling (early), possibly punched-out erosions (later).

DDx

- Septic arthritis
- Pseudogout
- Acute flare of osteoarthritis (most common condition that affects the 1st MTP)
- Cellulitis

According to ACR/EULAR guidelines gout can also be clinically diagnosed (joint/tophi aspiration unavailable) if a score of ≥8 points. This is based upon:

- Pattern of joint involvement: ankle or midfoot (+1), 1st MTP joint (+2)
- Number of characteristics (one (+1), two (+2), three (+3)): erythema on joint, painful to touch/pressure, difficulty with walking / joint use
- Number of episodes: one episode (+1), recurrent episodes (+2)
- Tophus: present (+4)
- Serum urate: (mM/L) <0.24 (–4), <0.36 (0), <0.48 (+2), <60 (+3), >60 (+4)
- Fluid analysis for MSU of joint: –ve (–2), +ve (definitive diagnosis)
- Imaging evidence of urate deposition on USS: present (+4)
- Imaging evidence of gout-related joint damage on X-ray: present (+4)

Rapid onset of pain (maximum <24h), erythema over joint, and associated cardiovascular disease are also suggestive features but not included in scoring.

Management

- Confirm the diagnosis of gout and exclude other conditions, especially septic arthritis.
- The management of gout can be principally divided into prevention and treatment of acute attacks of gout (*Table 2.7.2*).
- Risk factors for chronic hyperuricaemia and comorbidities should be identified and addressed.

Table 2.7.2: Management and prevention of gout in accordance with NICE NG219 (2022)

Management of acute gout	
NSAIDs	Prescribe as soon as possible and continue until 48 hours after the gout has resolved. Use 'strong' NSAIDs, e.g. indomethacin (50 mg/8 hours), or naproxen (0.5–1 g daily). Co-prescribe a PPI in high-risk individuals.
Colchicine	If NSAIDs are contraindicated, not tolerated, or have been ineffective in previous attacks, prescribe oral colchicine (0.5 mg/6 hours). Diarrhoea is a common side-effect.
Corticosteroids	• If NSAIDs and colchicine are contraindicated, e.g. in renal impairment, consider a short course of oral systemic corticosteroids (e.g. prednisolone 15 mg daily). • Intra-articular corticosteroids are an option if no more than 2 joints are affected.
Paracetamol	With/without codeine, in addition to above drugs or alone, solely for pain relief.
IL-1 inhibitor	Should only be used if NSAIDs, colchicine and corticosteroids are not tolerated / contraindicated / ineffective. Examples of IL-1 inhibitors used are anakinra and canakinumab. Current infection is a contraindication for use.
Prevention of gout	
Lifestyle changes	↓ Body weight, ↓ excessive consumption of food rich in purines (meat and seafood), ↓ alcohol, take regular exercise and stop smoking.
Allopurinol (xanthine oxidase inhibitor (XOi))	• Start allopurinol (100 mg OD) 1–2 weeks after inflammation has settled and titrate the dose, aiming for a serum uric acid of <360 μmol/L. • A lower target uric acid level <300 μmol/L may be considered for patients who have tophi, chronic gouty arthritis or continue to have ongoing frequent flares despite having a uric acid <360 μmol/L. • Co-prescribe a low-dose NSAID, or low-dose colchicine, for 3–6 months to prevent acute attacks of gout. Avoid stopping allopurinol in subsequent acute attacks once established on treatment. If prior allergic response and no other ULT agent can be used then allopurinol desensitization can be trialled with caution.
Febuxostat (XOi)	Consider as second-line therapy if allopurinol is contraindicated / not tolerated.
Uricase (urate oxidase) agents	May be used in specific cases as an adjunct to XOi if there is suboptimal control having trialled 2 XOi monotherapies. Pegloticase is an example which can be given as an infusion every 2 weeks.

Self-assessment

A 55 year old obese male complains of a sudden onset painful, red and swollen big toe. A diagnosis of crystal arthritis is strongly suspected.

1. Which conditions would you consider in your differential diagnosis? Name the most important one and state why.
2. What are the typical clinical features of an attack of acute gout?
3. What risk factors predispose the patient to gout?
4. A joint aspiration is performed. How would you examine the aspirate and what results would you expect?
5. Name two treatments for acute gout. What are the common side-effects of these medications?
6. What dietary advice would you provide to the patient?
7. Name two medications that can be started to prevent further attacks of gout.

Answers to self-assessment questions are to be found on the Resources tab at www.scionpublishing.com/Rheum2.

2.8 Calcium pyrophosphate disease

Calcium pyrophosphate disease (CPPD), often referred to as **pseudogout**, is caused by the shedding of **calcium pyrophosphate crystals** into the **joint space**. CPPD is commonly idiopathic; however, it can coexist with other conditions, often **osteoarthritis**, and is a very common cause of **chondrocalcinosis** (**calcification of cartilage** seen on X-ray).

Pathophysiology

- **Calcium pyrophosphate (CPP) crystals** form **extracellularly** when **inorganic pyrophosphate** (originating from the breakdown of ATP) reacts with **calcium**.
- There may be increased levels of pyrophosphate due to a **mutation in the *ANKH* gene**.
- The crystals are first deposited in the joint **cartilage** (**fibrocartilage** and **hyaline cartilage**) and then shed into the synovial fluid which can result in **inflammation** and later damage to the cartilage and surrounding tissue.
- This deposition can result in **chondrocalcinosis**.
- Age-related biochemical changes may encourage CPP crystal formation.
- **Hereditary and metabolic abnormalities** may lead to CPPD and it is most common in patients presenting under the age of 50.

Epidemiology and risk factors

- The prevalence of **CPPD** is ~**7–10%** in the **UK in people >60**.
- Men and women are equally affected.
- Mainly affects elderly, with CPPD prevalence in articular cartilage **doubling with each decade >60**.

Table 2.8.1: Risk factors for CPPD

Age >40 years	Trauma / injury
Osteoarthritis	Hyperparathyroidism
Hypomagnesaemia	Diuretics
Wilson's disease	Haemochromatosis
Hypothyroidism	Acromegaly

Clinical features

- May be **asymptomatic** but picked up on routine X-ray.
- Acute **tender, red, hot, swollen joint** suggests **acute CPPD** (also known as **pseudogout**). Episodes tend to last longer than gout.
- **Pain** and **stiffness** with long-term damage to joints (usually **knees**, **wrists**, **hips**, **and shoulders**) suggests **chronic CPPD**.
- **Polyarticular arthritic pattern** is most common for chronic CPPD. This may be distinguished from OA by level of joint damage in joints that are atypical for OA.

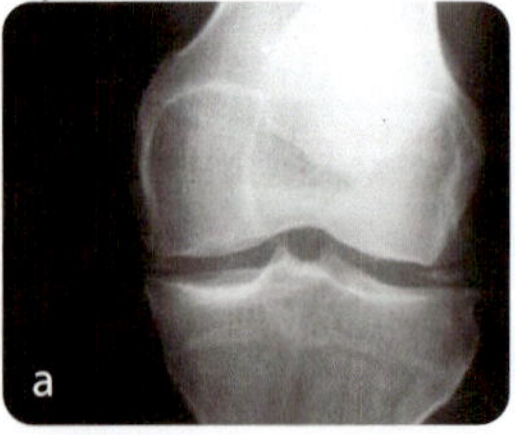

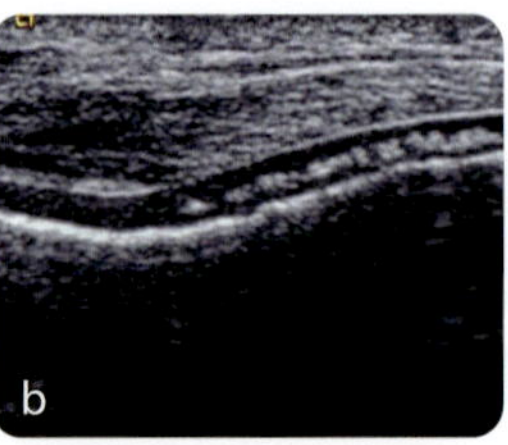

Fig. 2.8.1: (a) Plain X-ray showing CPP deposition in the fibrocartilage of the knee (chondrocalcinosis). **(b)** Ultrasound of the knee showing similar deposition.

OSCE tips: Gout vs CPPD

Gout	CPPD
Negatively birefringent crystals under polarized light microscopy	Positively birefringent crystals under polarized light microscopy
Deposition of monosodium urate crystals	Deposition of CPP crystals
Typically affects 1st MTP; ankle and mid-tarsal joints are also commonly affected	Typically affects larger joints, e.g. knee, wrist and ankle
More common in men	Equal sex distribution
Presentation is similar for both acute gout and acute CPPD, but there is usually a difference in joint distribution	
Acute management for both conditions is very similar (NSAIDs and colchicine); allopurinol has no role in the prevention of CPPD	

Diagnosis and investigations

Hx

- **Severe joint pain** and **swelling** that reaches its maximum within **6–24 weeks** is likely to be acute crystal inflammation, though this is not specific for acute CPP crystal arthritis.
- **Risk factors** (*Table 2.8.1*).

Ex

- **Large joints** affected, e.g. knee.
- **Tenderness** and **erythema**.
- **Signs** of the **underlying cause**, e.g. **osteoarthritis**.

Ix

- **Blood tests**: ↑ WCC, ↑ ESR, ↑ CRP (acute attack).
- **Joint X-rays**: chondrocalcinosis (*Fig. 2.8.1a*) and changes of OA.
- **Ultrasound**: (*Fig. 2.8.1b*). Can also be used to aid joint aspiration.
- **Aspiration of the joint and synovial fluid analysis**: ↑ WCC. Positive birefringent rhomboid-shaped crystals (i.e. CPP crystals) under polarized light microscopy. The joint fluid may appear purulent in nature.

DDx

- Septic arthritis
- Gout
- Osteoarthritis (chronic CPPD)
- Cellulitis

ACR/EULAR guidance allows diagnosis to be made if there is crowded dense syndrome or evidence of CPP crystals on joint aspiration. It can also be diagnosed if a score of >56 is achieved based on the following criteria:

- Age at symptom onset: >60 (+4).
- Time course and symptoms of inflammatory arthritis: persistent inflammatory arthritis (+9), one typical acute episode (+12), >1 typical acute episode (+16).
- Site of episode (score highest): first MTP (–6), joints other than those listed (+5), wrist (+8), knee (+9).
- Metabolic disease (see *Table 2.8.1*): present (+6).
- Synovial fluid analysis: absent on 2 occasions (–7), absent on one occasion (–1), present (+ve diagnosis).
- OA on imaging: OA of radiocarpal joints bilaterally (+2), >2 of the following findings: STT joint OA without first CMC joint OA, second MCP joint OA, third MCP joint OA (+7).
- Imaging evidence of CPPD (USS, CT or DECT): none (–4), present (+16).
- Number of joints with imaging evidence of CPPD: one (+16), two–three (+23), four or more (+25).

Management

- Any underlying causes need to be managed appropriately.
- Optimal treatment requires both non-pharmacological and pharmacological treatments.
  - **Non-pharmacological management** – initial rest followed by gradual mobilization of the joint. **Ice packs** may have a role in the short term for symptom relief.
  - **Pharmacological management** – **NSAIDs**, **colchicine**, intra-articular injection of long-acting **corticosteroids**. Adrenocorticotrophic hormone has shown some promise in treating acute CPPD if glucocorticosteroids are not tolerated; however, this is not well researched. This is the same for methotrexate and IL-1 inhibitors.

2.9 Vasculitis

Vasculitides (singular, vasculitis) are a heterogeneous group of diseases that are categorized by inflammation of blood vessels, leading to compromise of the vascular lumen and ischaemia. The commonest form of vasculitis is **giant cell arteritis** (**GCA**; see *Sec. 2.10*). Other less common vasculitides include **Takayasu's arteritis**, **polyarteritis nodosa (PAN)**, **granulomatosis with polyangiitis (GPA)**, also known as Wegener's granulomatosis (WG), **Churg–Strauss syndrome (CSS)** and **Henoch–Schönlein purpura (HSP)**.

Pathophysiology

Vasculitides may affect small, medium or large vessels (mainly arterial vessels).

Disease aetiology can be classified into either:

- **Primary** (idiopathic), which are autoimmune disorders (usually developed by exposure to some antigen) and account for 45–55% of vasculitides (*Fig. 2.9.1*).
- **Secondary**, mainly due to:
  - **infection** (15–20%) such as hepatitis B and C, TB and syphilis
  - **connective tissue disease** (15–20%) such as SLE, mixed connective tissue disease (MCTD) and RA
  - **drugs** (10–15%) e.g. hydralazine, propylthiouracil, sulphonamides, beta-lactams and quinolones.

There are several factors (genetics, environment, and abnormalities in immune response) which lead to vasculitis, and the pathology may vary between them. However, there are three suggested mechanisms.

- **Pathogenic immune complex formation (PIC)**
  - Antigen–antibody complexes are formed and deposited in vessel walls made more permeable by histamines, and bradykinin (released by mast cells).
  - This leads to the activation of complement (C5a) which attracts neutrophils into the vessel walls. These damage the wall through the release of enzymes which in turn recruits monocytes, compromising the lumen further and the process becomes chronic.
  - Many patients with vasculitis do not have detectable immune complexes deposited and the causal role is poorly understood.
- **Antineutrophil cytoplasmic antibodies (ANCA)**
  - ANCA target enzyme proteins in the cytoplasmic granules of neutrophils and monocytes. They are either c-ANCA (targeting proteinase-3) or p-ANCA (targeting myeloperoxidase).
  - In activated neutrophils and monocytes these enzymes become accessible to extracellular ANCA. ANCA causes neutrophil degranulation and the release of reactive oxygen species which can destroy endothelial cells and release pro-inflammatory cytokines (IL-1/8).
  - However, this may not be a primary pathogenesis, as antibody titres do not correlate with disease severity.
- **Pathogenic T lymphocyte response and granuloma formation (PTLG)**
  - Vascular endothelial cells express HLA (II) after activation by cytokines (IFN-γ) like antigen-presenting macrophages. They can also produce IL-1 which activates T cells.
  - This starts immunological processes within the vessel, and further adhesion molecules are propagated. This recruits more leucocytes to the endothelial cells, resulting in inflammation and compromise.

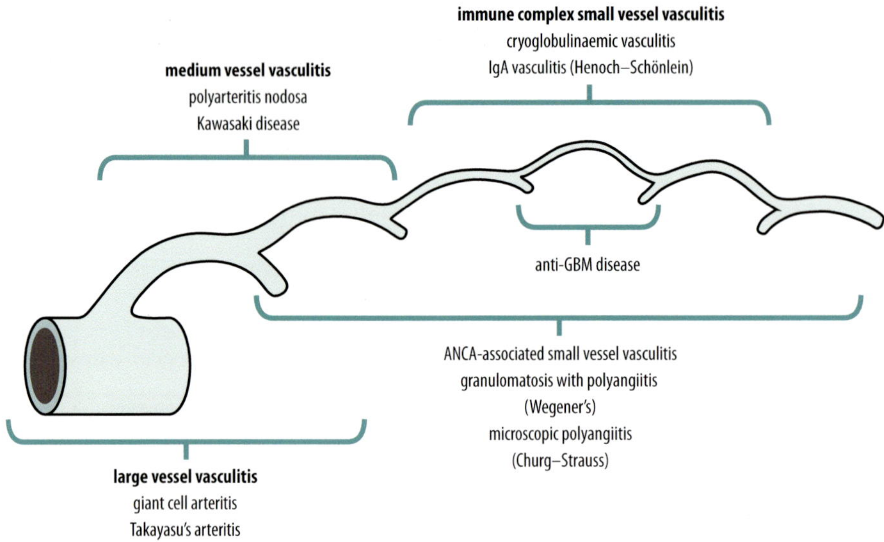

Fig. 2.9.1: Vasculitis classification. International Chapel Hill Consensus Conference Nomenclature of Vasculitides (CHCC 2012).

Table 2.9.1: Classification of vasculitis

Category	Condition	Definition
Large arteries	**Giant cell arteritis (GCA)**	Discussed in *Sec. 2.10.*
	Takayasu's arteritis	Granulomatous inflammation of the large arteries supplying the arm, head, neck and heart, leading to aortic arch syndrome. Occurs mainly in young women. **Potential mechanism: PTLG**
Medium arteries	**Polyarteritis nodosa (PAN)**	PAN is **necrotizing arteritis** without **glomerulonephritis** and is not associated with ANCA. This can lead to aneurysm, thrombosis and infarction. Poor prognosis with death often being GI-related.
Small arteries (c-ANCA and/or p-ANCA +ve)	**Granulomatosis with polyangiitis (Wegener's)**	A **necrotizing vasculitis** which is usually associated with **granulomatous inflammation** of the **respiratory tract** and glomerulonephritis. **Potential mechanism: ANCA** The pathological hallmarks of WG are chronic granulomatous inflammation and vasculitis. They are typically c-ANCA (+) during active disease and are at an increased risk of thrombotic events.

Table 2.9.1: Classification of vasculitis *(continued)*

Category	Condition	Definition
Small arteries (p-ANCA +ve)	**Churg–Strauss syndrome (CSS)**	Eosinophil-rich and necrotizing granulomatous inflammation associated with asthma and eosinophilia. **Potential mechanism: ANCA + PTLG**
	Microscopic polyangiitis (MPA)	Necrotizing vasculitis causing glomerulonephritis. Pulmonary capillaritis is common. **Potential mechanism: ANCA**
Small arteries (ANCA –ve)	**Anti-glomerular basement membrane (GBM) disease**	Vasculitis affecting glomerular capillaries, pulmonary capillaries, or both, with deposition of anti-basement membrane autoantibodies.
Immune complex small vessel vasculitis	**Henoch–Schönlein purpura (HSP)**	IgA dominant immune deposition. Usually affects the skin and GI tract and frequently causes arthritis. **Potential mechanism: PIC**
Variable vessel vasculitis	**Behçet's syndrome**	Vasculitis that can affect arteries or veins, although mainly venules. Thrombosis is associated with it and it has a relapsing course. Almost any organ can be affected. Common in those of Turkish descent, and very rare in the UK.

Epidemiology and risk factors

- Vasculitis is a rare condition.
- Epidemiology varies, depending on the gender, the subtype of vasculitis and the geographical location.

Table 2.9.2: Risk factors for vasculitis

Other disorders	• RA and SLE can cause secondary vasculitis. • A history of **asthma and/or nasal allergies** is associated with CSS.
Age	• WG and CSS occur mainly in those aged >40. • HSP occurs mainly in children and young adults.
Gender	• Large vessel vasculitis is more common in women. • PAN affects men more than women.
Infection	• Syphilis, TB and hepatitis B and C are associated with secondary vasculitis.
Ethnicity	• Many forms of vasculitis are more common in Caucasian patients compared to other ethnicities. • Behçet's disease is more common in those of Turkish descent.
Geographical and environmental factors	• WG is more common amongst northern Europeans and commonly presents in winter following respiratory infection. • Microscopic polyangiitis is more common in southern Europe.

Clinical features

Takayasu's arteritis

Commonly divided into two stages:

1. **Systemic stage** (due to inflammation of artery prior to occlusion): non-specific symptoms such as fever, malaise, fatigue, weight loss and arthralgia.
2. **Occlusive stage:**
    - Usually presents with claudication of the arm.
    - Loss of arm pulses, variation in blood pressure >10 mmHg between arms.
    - Arterial bruits over any large artery.
    - Aortic regurgitation (approx. 20%).
    - Often associated with hypertension (most common presentation in children).

Polyarteritis nodosa (PAN)

- Presents with ischaemia or infarction within affected organs:
    - **GI tract** – abdominal pain, bleeding or perforation
    - **Heart** – angina or MI
    - **Kidneys** – hypertension and renal failure
    - **Peripheral nerves** – mononeuritis multiplex (due to inflammation of vessels supplying the nerve)
- Other presentations include weight loss, fever, raised diastolic blood pressure (>90 mmHg) and livedo reticularis (*Fig. 2.9.2*).
- PAN is common secondary to hepatitis B virus (HBV) infection.

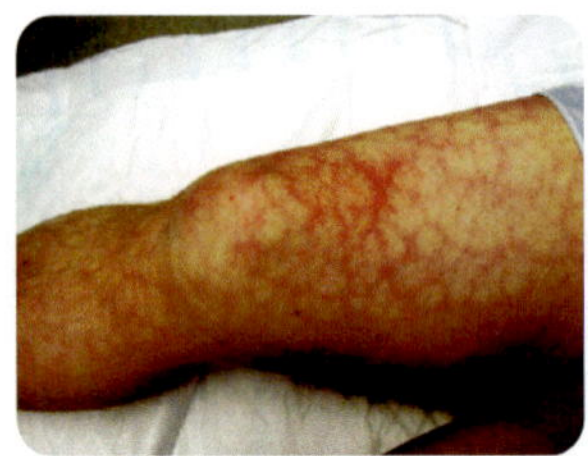

Fig. 2.9.2: Livedo reticularis on the anterior surface of the thigh.

Granulomatosis with polyangiitis, also known as Wegener's granulomatosis (WG)

A typical presentation involves the upper respiratory tract, lungs and kidneys:

- **Upper airway (90%) 'NOSE'**
    - **N**asal: obstruction and crusting, with rhinorrhoea, hyposmia, epistaxis, nasal septal perforation and saddle nose deformity (*Fig. 2.9.3*)
    - **O**cular: epiphora (watering eye) due to involvement of the nasolacrimal duct and lacrimal sac, scleritis/episcleritis (52%)
    - **S**inusitis and subglottic stenosis (hoarseness of voice is a classical feature observed in WG)
    - **E**ar: otitis media (recurrent), hearing loss, ear pain.
- **Pulmonary involvement (85%)**
    - A common radiological feature is the presence of single or multiple **cavitary nodules** (*Fig. 2.9.4*) at cortical and sub-pleural sites
    - This can manifest as a persistent cough (usually unproductive), pyrexia, haemoptysis, dyspnoea and post-obstructive infection.

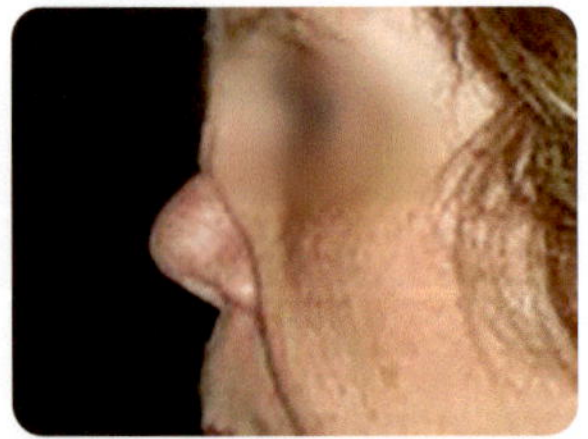

Fig. 2.9.3: Saddle nose deformity.

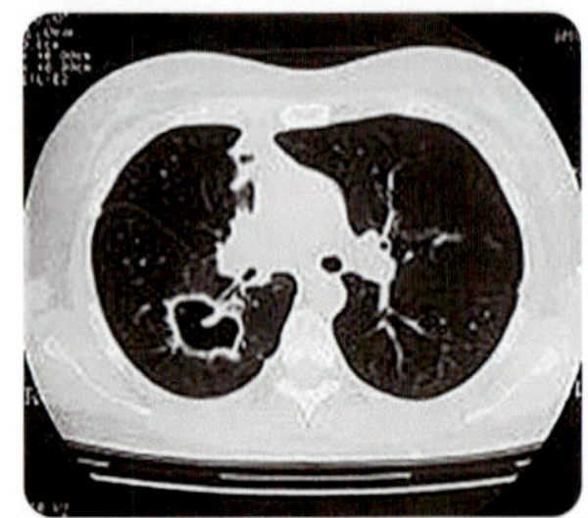

Fig. 2.9.4: Cavitary WG nodule in the right lung.

- **Kidneys (77%)**
  - Nephritic syndrome ('**PHAROH**'): **P**roteinuria, **H**aematuria, **A**zotaemia/uraemia, **R**ed blood cell casts, **O**liguria, **H**ypertension.

Other clinical features include skin rash (palpable purpura) (46%), conjunctival haemorrhages and scleritis.

Churg–Strauss syndrome

- Classically presents with skin lesions (purpura or nodules) (51%) and mononeuritis multiplex (72%) with asthma.
- Rhinitis and sinusitis (61%).
- 50% have abdominal pain due to mesenteric arteritis.

Microscopic polyangiitis (MPA)

- Shares many similarities with WG. Classically presents with rapidly progressive glomerulonephritis and sometimes alveolar haemorrhage (haemoptysis first sign).
- Common symptoms include tiredness, loss of appetite, myalgia and arthralgia.

Anti-glomerular basement membrane (GBM) disease

- Usually presents as part of the classic Goodpasture's syndrome.
- Goodpasture's syndrome is defined by the triad of anti-GBM antibodies, glomerulonephritis and pulmonary haemorrhage.

Henoch–Schönlein purpura (HSP)

- Typically presents with palpable purpuric rash (small raised reddish / purple bumps; *Fig. 2.9.5*) over buttocks and lower leg.
- Colicky abdominal pain and asymmetrical arthritis following upper respiratory tract infection.
- Glomerulonephritis occurs in 40% of patients, manifesting as proteinuria and haematuria.

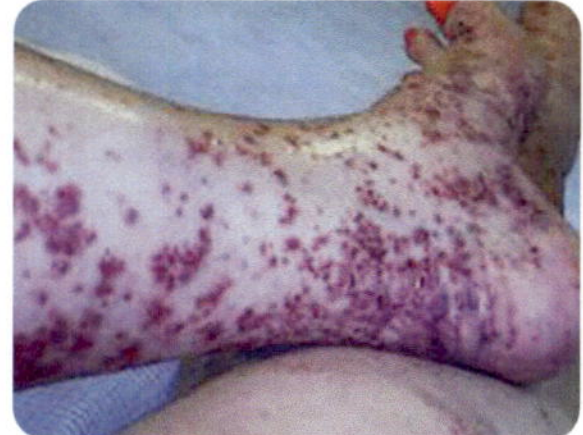
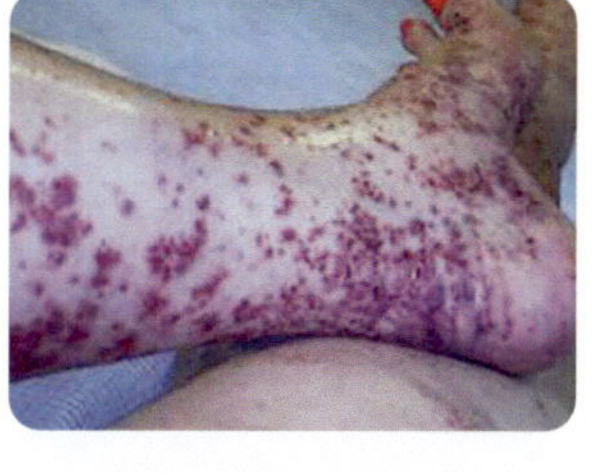

Fig. 2.9.5: Purpuric rash.

Behçet's disease

Behçet's disease is a systemic vasculitis of unknown cause. Typical presentation includes:

- Oral ulceration (*Fig. 2.9.6*)
- Genital ulceration
- Ocular involvement (anterior and posterior uveitis or retinal vascular lesions) (50%)
- Cutaneous lesions (including erythema nodosum or papulopustular rash)

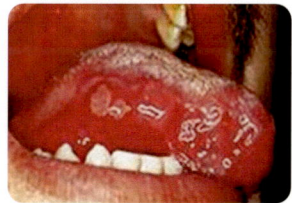

Fig. 2.9.6: Oral ulceration.

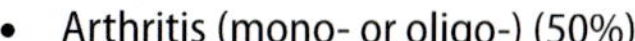

- Arthritis (mono- or oligo-) (50%)
- GI features, including diarrhoea and anorexia. Typically presents similarly to Crohn's.
- Neurological features, including encephalitis, confusion or cranial nerve palsy (5%).

Diagnosis and investigations

Hx

- Secondary vasculitis → any connective tissue disorders, recent infection and drug history.
- Ask about asthma and recent blood transfusions (HBV).

Ex

General examination

- **Skin**:
  - Palpable purpura – HSP, WG, CSS
  - Nodules, papules, ulcers, digital ischaemia – PAN
  - Vesiculobullous (blisters) lesion – CSS, HSP
  - Pallor – seen in any vasculitis
  - Splinter haemorrhages (under the nail)
- **Blood pressure**:
  - Hypertension – PAN, Takayasu's
- **Oral cavity**:
  - Strawberry tongue, lip cracking, congestion of oropharyngeal mucosa – Kawasaki syndrome
  - Strawberry gums, gum ulceration – WG
  - Oral ulcers – hallmark of Behçet's disease
- **Other**:
  - *Nose*: septal perforation, saddle nose deformity, mucosal ulceration – WG
  - *Pulse*: unequal pulse between left and right sides – Takayasu's arteritis
  - *Criteria*: International Study Group criteria for Behçet's disease (2014) Recurrent oral ulcers and 2 of genital ulcers, skin lesions, eye lesions, pathergy (+)

Systematic examination

Respiratory system: asthma – CSS
CVS: congestive heart failure – CSS
GI: abdominal tenderness (mesenteric ischaemia) – PAN
MSK: migratory polyarthritis – WG, CSS, MPA

Ix

Blood tests:

- **FBC**: normocytic anaemia; leucocytosis (e.g. eosinophilia), thrombocytosis (primary vasculitis); leucopenia or thrombocytopenia (secondary vasculitis)
- High eosinophil count (eosinophilia), and p-ANCA (+) for CSS (48%)
- **Electrolytes**: hyperkalaemia in renal failure
- Raised **creatinine** in renal failure
- LFT abnormal in hepatitis B or C (may need to test for serology to confirm / rule out)

Immunology:

- Presence of c-ANCA and anti-proteinase 3 (anti-PR3) is very specific (>90%) for WG
- Presence of p-ANCA and anti-MPO is seen in MPA and CSS

Urine dipstick (glomerulonephritis)

Imaging:

- CXR (lung involvement) and echocardiogram (cardiac abnormalities)
- Angiography: look for aneurysms, stenosis and post-stenotic dilatations in Takayasu's and PAN
- CT/MRI angiography: look at aorta and major branches (Takayasu's)
- Ultrasound (± Doppler enhancement): readily available and non-invasive. Preferred in early or mild disease and children (Takayasu's)

Biopsy of the suspected vessel:

- Commonly taken from the site where vasculitis is suspected; e.g. temporal artery, nasal mucosa, sinuses and skin

Skin pathergy test:

- Performed when Behçet's syndrome suspected (very specific)
- Needleprick leads to papule formation within 48 hrs

DDx

- Primary vasculitis
- Secondary vasculitis
- Peripheral vascular disease, e.g. venous thromboembolism
- Antiphospholipid syndrome

Management

General principles:

- Treat any associated disease and remove any identified precipitating antigen.
- Level of treatment aggression should relate to how likely a disease may progress to irreversible end-organ damage.
- **Induce remission**; this can be achieved by **high-dose steroids** and/or **cyclophosphamide/ rituximab** (both orally and intravenously, depending on symptoms and diagnosis).

- Once remission is induced, the dose of steroid is **gradually reduced** and a **steroid-sparing agent** such as **methotrexate**, **tocilizumab** or **azathioprine** is started.
- The patient is **maintained** on **low-dose steroids** and a steroid-sparing agent whilst being actively monitored.
- Additional therapies include angioplasty, plasma exchange and biological agents such as an IL-6 inhibitor.
- Supportive therapy such as analgesia and anti-inflammatory drugs, and prophylactic therapy (commonly trimethoprim-sulfamethoxazole) are given when needed.
- Vascular surgery intervention should be considered if there are disease stigmata present, such as limb claudication.

Self-assessment

A 35 year old woman presents with recurrent otitis media. She has a history of numerous episodes of epistaxis. On examination you notice that she has a prominent saddle nose, dark crusts in her nose and diminished hearing. Nasal mucosal biopsy shows granulomata and large areas of necrosis.

1. What is the most likely diagnosis?
2. What specific autoantibodies are associated with this disease?
3. What other signs and symptoms may she have?
4. What is the pharmacological agent of choice for this condition?

Answers to self-assessment questions are to be found on the Resources tab at www.scionpublishing.com/Rheum2.

2.10 Giant cell arteritis

Giant cell arteritis (GCA), also known as temporal arteritis, is one of the most common forms of vasculitis, typically affecting the **temporal artery**. It is closely associated with polymyalgia rheumatica and affects medium- and large-sized vessels. It needs early recognition and treatment to minimize the risk of complications such as permanent loss of vision.

Pathophysiology

- GCA is an autoimmune disorder, where exposure to an unknown environmental trigger (possibly an infectious agent) causes breakdown of immune tolerance, resulting in an autoimmune reaction against the arterial wall.
- T cells infiltrate the arterial wall through the vasa vasorum and activate macrophage differentiation. They chiefly produce IFN-γ and IL-2, IL- 6 pro-inflammatory cytokines.
- GCA mainly affects the **extra-cranial branches** of the **carotid artery**, specifically the **temporal artery**. However, it can affect any branch of the aorta. Patients typically have vasculitis of multiple vessels, which can be difficult to detect.
- The histopathological hallmark of GCA is the predominance of mononuclear infiltrates or granulomas, usually with **multinucleated giant cells**.
- Inflammatory cells stimulate the release of metalloproteases (MMPs) and reactive oxygen species (ROS) which damage the extracellular matrix of the blood vessel wall.

Epidemiology and risk factors

- GCA is the most common vasculitis in the UK, with an incidence of about 2.2 per 10 000 person years.

Table 2.10.1: Risk factors for primary vasculitis

Polymyalgia rheumatica	• 50% of patients with GCA have PMR. This more commonly presents after GCA.
Age	• GCA occurs almost exclusively in patients >50 years old.
Gender	• GCA is 2–3 × more common in females.
Ethnicity	• Mainly affects Caucasians.

Clinical features

- Abrupt-onset **headache**, usually unilateral in the temporal area.
- **Scalp pain** (50%).
- Temporal artery **tenderness** and **swelling** (*Fig. 2.10.1*) with loss of pulsation in some cases.
- **Visual symptoms**, due to ophthalmic artery involvement, are a very serious complication of GCA (up to 30% of patients). Specific symptoms of visual involvement should always be asked. These should not be missed and include:
    - **Amaurosis fugax** (transient loss of vision in one eye)
    - Blurring and diplopia
    - Partial or complete loss of vision

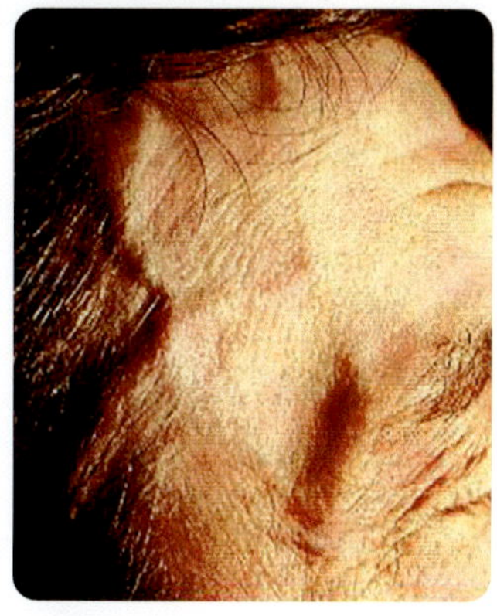

Fig. 2.10.1: Swollen temporal artery in GCA patient.

- **Jaw** and **tongue claudication (~50%)**
- **Neurological symptoms** (mono/poly peripheral neuropathy, upper cranial nerve palsy) (30%)
- Systemic features of PMR commonly include: fever, fatigue, weight loss and muscle aching.

Diagnosis and investigations

Hx

- Ask about onset of headache and whether one-sided (often in temporal or occipital region, worse at night and when touching scalp).
- Ask about whether they have polymyalgia rheumatica (PMR) or PMR symptoms.
- Ask about visual symptoms (amaurosis fugax, diplopia, and partial or complete loss of vision).
- Patient might complain of jaw claudication ('Painful jaw when chewing?').

Ex

Vascular:

- Scalp tenderness
- Tenderness of temporal artery and/or decreased temporal artery pulse
- Carotid bruits might be heard on auscultation
- Abdominal bruits or abnormal pulsatile aneurysmal swelling

Examination of the eye and vision:

- Ophthalmoscopic examination may reveal pale optic disc associated with severe loss of vision acuity
- Referral to ophthalmologist to perform slit-lamp examination may be required.

Ix

Blood tests:

- ↑ ESR ≥50 mm/hour.
- **CRP** often elevated.
- FBC → normocytic, normochromic anaemia, thrombocytosis.

Biopsy of the suspected vessel:

- Biopsy of the involved vessel may show a typical appearance of intermittent inflammation ('skip lesions'), or it may even be negative (20–30%). Biopsy should be a long segment (>1 cm) and within 2 weeks of starting oral glucocorticosteroids (GCS).

Imaging:

- Ultrasound may reveal thickening of the affected blood vessel wall ('halo sign').
- MRI (temporal/extracranial) has similar diagnostic value to biopsy.

DDx

- Migraine
- Tension headache
- Trigeminal neuralgia

Rapid diagnosis box: The ACR/EULAR classification criteria for GCA (2022)

1. **Age** at disease onset ≥50 years (absolute requirement).
2. **New headache** (localized pain in the head), **morning stiffness** (shoulders/neck), **claudication** (jaw/tongue), **scalp tenderness, bilateral axillary involvement on imaging,** and **fluorodeoxyglucose-PET activity throughout aorta** (+2 each).
3. **Temporal artery abnormality** (vascular examination) (+2).
4. **Elevated ESR** (≥50 mm/hour) or **CRP** (≥10 mg/L) (+3).
5. **Abnormal artery biopsy** – mononuclear cell infiltration or granulomatous inflammation, usually with multinucleated giant cells), or halo sign on USS (+5).
6. **Sudden visual loss** (+3).

For purposes of classification, a patient has giant cell (temporal) arteritis if a score of six or more is achieved.

Management

- Immediate initiation of **high-dose glucocorticoid** treatment after clinical suspicion of GCA is raised.
- Visual loss occurs early in the course of disease and is irreversible.
- Early treatment with high-dose glucocorticoid is essential to prevent any further visual deterioration.

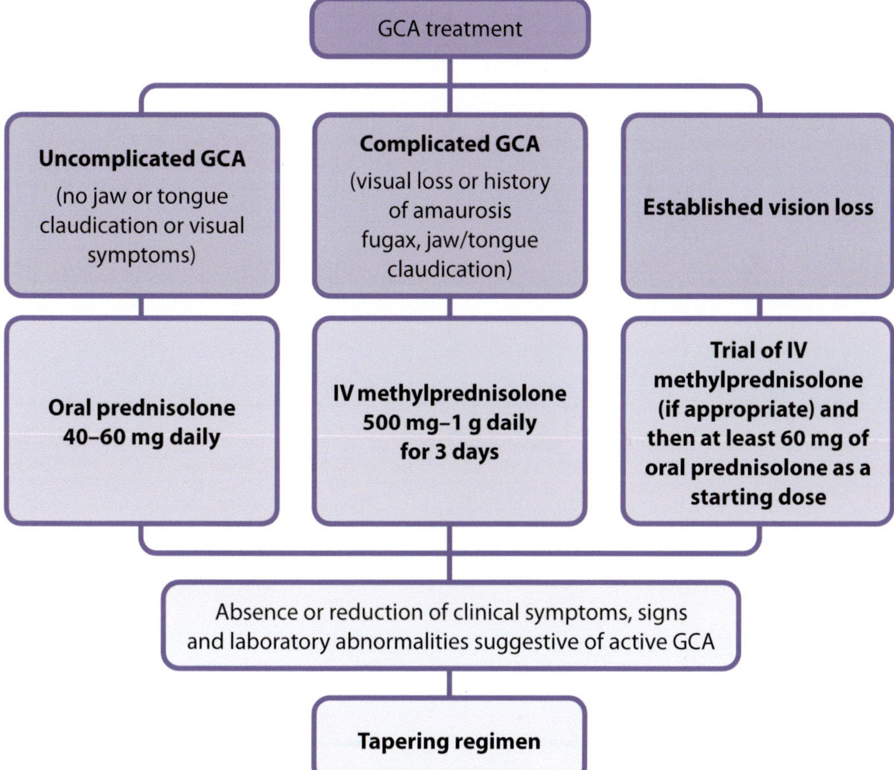

Fig. 2.10.2: Overview of GCA management (*Adapted from the British Society of Rheumatology*).

- Bone protection, such as a **bisphosphonate** and **calcium / vitamin D supplementation**, should be strongly considered.
- Tapering regimen: 40–60 mg prednisolone continued for 4 weeks. Then reduce dose by 10 mg every 2 weeks to 20 mg. Then by 2.5 mg every 2–4 weeks to 10 mg. Then by 1 mg every 1–2 months (provided there is no relapse). Tocilizumab/methotrexate can be considered as an adjunct to tapering therapy in patients who relapse or are at risk of glucocorticoid toxicity.
- Surgical advice should be sought if there are worsening signs of limb ischaemia.
- Long-term monitoring is required once GCA is in remission (FBC, ESR/CRP) and adverse effects of corticosteroids.

Self-assessment

A 60 year old female presents with partial vision loss in her left eye. She complains of bitemporal headache for several weeks, along with pain and stiffness in the neck and shoulders. There are also signs of low grade fever, fatigue and weight loss. On physical examination, there is tenderness of the scalp over the temporal areas as well as thickening of the temporal arteries.

1. What is the most likely diagnosis?
2. What medication should be immediately administered?
3. Why may this patient have stiffness in the neck and shoulders?
4. What specific blood test would you request?
5. What more specific investigations can be used to try to confirm the diagnosis?

Answers to self-assessment questions are to be found on the Resources tab at www.scionpublishing.com/Rheum2.

2.11 Polymyalgia rheumatica

Polymyalgia rheumatica (PMR) is an **inflammatory condition** that results in **muscle pain** and stiffness in the **shoulder** and **pelvic girdle. Giant cell arteritis (GCA)** is a more serious condition which usually coexists with PMR. This association is so strong that PMR and GCA might be conditions on the spectrum of the same disease; however, each can exist in isolation.

Pathophysiology

- The cause is unknown, but an ageing immune system may play a role; genetic polymorphisms and environmental factors contribute to disease susceptibility.
- A viral cause hypothesis has been suggested for PMR and GCA (e.g. adenovirus, respiratory syncytial virus, human parainfluenza virus), but this has not been confirmed.
- IL-6 production is increased in PMR patients and a large increase in monocytes and neutrophils (myeloid shift) is seen.
- ↓ B-cell numbers in newly diagnosed PMR patients have been noted. This may imply a regulatory mechanism for B cells in the pathogenesis of PMR.
- Association of HLA-DRB1*04 and -DRB1*01 alleles has been reported in various population studies, e.g. in Northern European descent.
- **Inflammation** is central to the pathogenesis of PMR, and **synovial thickening** and inflammation may be seen in arthroscopy.

Epidemiology and risk factors

- The incidence of the disease in patients over 40 is around 95.5 per 100 000 in the UK.
- The prevalence of PMR is around 0.85% in the UK.
- PMR is mainly seen in people of **north European** ancestry.

Table 2.11.1: Risk factors for PMR

Age	• Almost exclusively present in patients **over the age of 50**, with peak incidence at age 75.
Gender	• Female:male, **3:1**.
Giant cell arteritis	• Approximately 40–60% of those with GCA have PMR.
Genetics	• Having siblings with PMR increases the risk.

Clinical features

- **Bilateral shoulder** (90%) or **thigh muscle aching pain persisting** for **≥1 month**.
- **Morning stiffness** typically lasting for >45 min.
- Systemic features (~50%):
  - Loss of appetite
  - **Weight loss**
  - **Low grade malaise**
  - **Signs and symptoms of GCA** (*Sec. 2.10*)
  - Depression

- Peripheral MSK symptoms such as peripheral arthritis (asymmetric knees and wrists) (~50%).
- **It's important to exclude other conditions such as active infection, malignancy and GCA!**
- Main characteristic of PMR is the prompt **response to corticosteroids**.

ACR/EULAR PMR classification criteria (2012) (score of at least 4 required)

- **Age >50 years, bilateral shoulder pain and abnormal ESR/CRP**
- **Morning stiffness duration of >45 min** (+2)
- **Hip pain or limited range of motion** (+1)
- **Absence of RF or anti-CCP** (+2)
- **Absence of other joint pain** (+1)

Optional US criteria:

- At least **one shoulder** with **subdeltoid bursitis / biceps tenosynovitis / glenohumeral synovitis** and at least **one hip** with **synovitis / trochanteric bursitis** (+1)
- **Both shoulders** with **subdeltoid bursitis / biceps tenosynovitis / glenohumeral synovitis** (+1)

Diagnosis and investigations

Hx

- Presence of risk factors, e.g. age (>50 years).
- Acute onset shoulder / hip girdle pain and stiffness.
- Systemic features: low grade malaise, weight loss, depression.

Ex

- Normal muscle strength at initial presentation.
- There may be muscle tenderness proximally.
- **Temporal artery tenderness** suggests coexisting GCA.

Ix

Blood tests:

- Inflammatory markers:
  - **Raised ESR → >40 mm/hour**
  - Raised CRP

  NB: PMR may be diagnosed with a normal ESR/CRP if there are classical clinical features and response to steroids
  - Urea and electrolytes → kidney function
- Bone profile (calcium, alkaline phosphatase) → rule out bone disease.
- RA/anti-CCP → rule out RA.
- Creatine kinase → rule out myositis / muscle breakdown.
- Serum protein electrophoresis → measures **paraprotein level to exclude multiple myeloma**.
- Thyroid function test → **exclusion of thyroid diseases**.
- Radiography → exclusion of non-erosive joint disease.
- Urine for Bence Jones proteins → to rule out myeloma.
- Temporal artery biopsy → if GCA is clinically suspected.

DDx

- Polymyositis
- Metabolic bone, e.g. osteomalacia
- Hypothyroidism
- Elderly onset of RA
- Fibromyalgia
- Possible underlying malignancy, e.g. multiple myeloma

Management

- Start with standardized daily dose of 15–25 mg **prednisolone**. **Clinical response of >70% in one week** is expected in PMR. Inflammatory markers should ideally be normalized in 4 weeks.
- The dose of prednisolone is reduced gradually with the aim of stopping altogether. An example regime (NICE 2024) is: once symptoms are controlled to 12.5 mg/day for 3 weeks, it should then be reduced to 10 mg/day for 4–6 weeks then reduced by 1 mg/day every 4–8 weeks. If relapse occurs increase prednisolone dose to pre-relapse level and start reduction again when controlled.
- IM methylprednisolone can be considered as an alternative to oral prednisolone.
- Due to long-term use of steroids, bone protective agent (e.g. **bisphosphonate**) and gastroprotective agent (e.g. **proton pump inhibitor (PPI)**) should be used.
- Most treatment can be discontinued after 18–24 months.
- Steroid-sparing agents, such as methotrexate, azathioprine and tocilizumab, may also be used. Patients should be **monitored for the emergence of GCA**.
- If GCA occurs, then a higher initial prednisolone dose should be used (40–60 mg/day).
- Education about diet and control of other comorbidities should be given and a personalized exercise programme should be made to reduce the risk of falls and maintain muscle mass.

Self-assessment

A 56 year old female presents with a 4 week history of fatigue, weight loss, fevers, and bilateral pain and stiffness in the shoulder and hip girdles. She experiences difficulty getting out of bed in the morning due to stiffness, but these symptoms improve as the day progresses.

1. What is the most likely diagnosis? Give reasons for this.
2. What other condition is strongly linked to this diagnosis?
3. What investigations would you perform and why?
4. How should this patient be managed?

Answers to self-assessment questions are to be found on the Resources tab at www.scionpublishing.com/Rheum2.

2.12 Systemic lupus erythematosus

Systemic lupus erythematosus (SLE) is a **chronic multi-systemic autoimmune disease** of unknown cause that most commonly affects **women (90%)** during their **reproductive years**. Since it can affect any organ system, its presentation and course are highly variable. The disease is characterized by the presence of **antinuclear antibodies (ANA).** There are other types of lupus (other than systemic), for instance **discoid lupus**, **drug-induced lupus** and overlap syndromes.

Pathophysiology

Breakdown of self-tolerance

- Although the specific cause of SLE is unknown, multiple factors are associated with the development of the disease, including **genetic** (relationships between certain polymorphisms and clinical manifestations) and **environmental factors** such as **oxidative stress**, **infections** (possible EBV), **UV light exposure** and **drugs (drug-induced lupus)**. SLE occurs when there are enough risk variants present.
- Many **innate** and **acquired** immune disturbances occur in SLE, which eventually results in the development of **autoantibodies** and **autoreactive T-cells** (*Fig. 2.12.1*).

Activation of the innate immune system

- Leads to the production of **IFN-α** by dendritic cells. This leads to the upregulation of genes induced by IFN-α creating a hallmark 'genetic signature' of SLE (80%).
- Activated macrophages produce IL-12, TNF-α and B-cell maturation and survival factors.
- Defective clearance of **apoptotic cells**, **immune complexes**, and failure to produce factors needed for T regulatory cell production lead to persistently high levels of autoantigens.

Dysregulation of the adaptive immune system and autoantibody production

- The innate immune system also interacts with B and T cells of acquired immunity, leading to **hyperactivation by epigenetic modification**.
- Central B cells are, therefore, encouraged to secrete autoantibodies. The most common autoantibodies are antinuclear (**ANA**; 98%), **anti-dsDNA** (70%), **antierythrocyte** (60%) and **antineuronal** (60%).
- Autoantibody-secreting B cells are more prevalent in SLE patients, and their survival is encouraged by IL-6, 10, and oestrogen.
- **Antiphospholipid antibodies** are a specific family of autoantibodies directed against **anionic phospholipids** located in cell membranes (**antiphospholipid syndrome**, see *Box 2.12.2*).
- Abnormal elevations in calcium influx and cytokine production pathways result in less production of IL-2 (T lymphocyte survival and production of T regulatory cells) and overproduction of IL-17 (T helper cell production). This creates a defective suppressive network for immune complex formation.

Inflammation and tissue damage

- After the deposition of autoantibodies and immune complexes the **complement system** is activated and plays a major role in tissue damage.

- Inflammation activates tissue-fixed cells, resulting in sclerosis and fibrosis in multiple tissues. It also triggers the release of vasoactive peptides, reactive oxygen species (ROS) (causing oxidative damage), and growth factors.

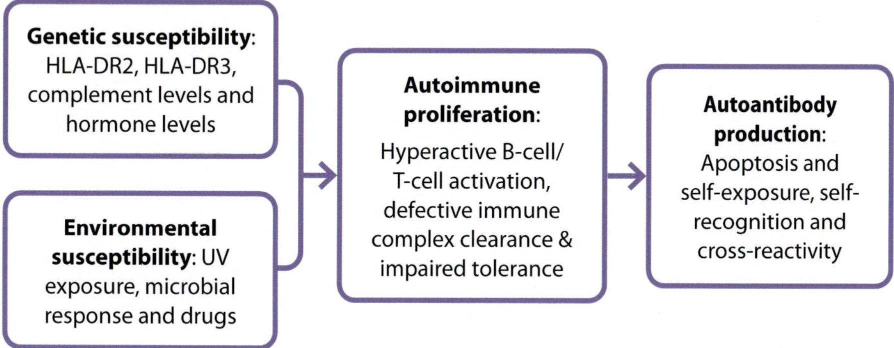

Fig. 2.12.1: Summary of pathogenesis of SLE.

Epidemiology and risk factors

- The prevalence of SLE is approximately 50 000 in the UK.
- The incidence of SLE is approximately 4 cases per 100 000 in the UK.

Table 2.12.1: Risk factors for SLE

Female sex	• The female to male ratio is approximately **10:1**.
Age	• The incidence increases in women of **childbearing age (15–45)**.
Ethnicity	• More common in **Afro-Caribbeans** and **Asians**.
Drugs	• **Minocycline**, **isoniazid**, **procainamide**, **quinidine**, **chlorpromazine** and **methyldopa** can cause drug-induced lupus.
Sun exposure	• May be an important environmental trigger of SLE.
Family history	• Genetic factors include **HLA-DR2/3**, **complement**, **Fc gamma receptor**, **cytotoxic T-lymphocyte antigen-4** and **cytokine genes**.
Tobacco smoking	• Smoking is linked not only to the development of SLE but also to the prognosis of the disease.

Clinical features

- SLE is a remitting and relapsing illness, typically presenting with non-specific constitutional symptoms of **malaise**, **fatigue**, **myalgia** and **fever**.
- See *Box 2.12.1* for specific features.
- Other features include **lymphadenopathy**, **weight loss**, **alopecia**, **nail-fold infarcts**, **non-infective endocarditis**, **Raynaud's**, **migraine**, **stroke**, and **retinal exudates**.

Box 2.12.1: The ACR/EULAR classification criteria (2019)

(+) ANA for criteria to be applied. If a score of 10 or more is achieved a classification of SLE can be made. Only the highest scoring criterion in each domain should be scored.

Fever >38°C (+2) and '**MS BRAIN**'

Mucocutaneous
- **Oral ulcers**: oral or nasopharyngeal ulceration, usually painless, observed by physician (+2)
- **Non-scarring alopecia** (+2)
- **Malar rash** (*Fig. 2.12.3*) **(acute cutaneous)**: fixed erythema, flat or raised, over the malar eminences, tending to spare the nasolabial folds (+6)
- **Discoid rash** (*Fig. 2.12.4*) / **subacute cutaneous**: erythematous raised patches with adherent keratotic scaling and follicular plugging; atrophic scarring may occur in older lesions (+4)

Serositis (one of the following):
- Pleuritis: convincing history of pleuritic pain, pleural rubs on auscultation, or evidence of pleural effusion (+5)
- Pericarditis: documented by ECG, pericardial rub, or evidence of pericardial effusion (+6)

Blood disorders (one of the following):
- Leucopenia: $<4 \times 10^9$/L (+3)
- Autoimmune haemolysis (+4)
- Thrombocytopenia: $<100\,000 \times 10^9$/L in the absence of offending drugs (+4)

Renal disorder:
- Persistent proteinuria >0.5 g/day (+4)
- Renal biopsy class II or V lupus nephritis (+8)
- Renal biopsy class III or IV lupus nephritis (+10)

Arthritis: non-erosive arthritis involving ≥2 peripheral joints, characterized by tenderness, swelling or effusion (+6)

Immunological disorder (one of the following):
- SLE-specific antibodies: anti-dsDNA: presence of antibody to native DNA in abnormal titre or anti-Smith: presence of antibody to Smith nuclear antigen (+6)
- Positive findings of antiphospholipid antibodies (anti-cardiolipin or lupus anticoagulant or anti-beta2 glycoprotein 1 antibodies) (+2)
- Low C3 **or** C4 (+3)
- Low C3 **and** C4 (+4)

Neurological disorder (one of the following):
- Delirium (+2)
- Psychosis: in the absence of offending drugs or known metabolic derangements, e.g. uraemia, ketoacidosis or electrolyte imbalance (+3)
- Seizures: in the absence of offending drugs or known metabolic derangements, e.g. uraemia, ketoacidosis, or electrolyte imbalance (+5)

Diagnosis and investigations

Hx
- **Clinical presentation** (*see above*)
- **Family history**
- **Drug history**
- Other risk factors – sun exposure and tobacco smoking.

Ex

Since any organ system can be affected in SLE, multiple organ systems need to be assessed (*Fig. 2.12.2*):

1. **Mucocutaneous**: painful / painless oral ulcers, malar rash, diffuse or patchy alopecia (*Fig. 2.12.5*) and photosensitivity (common), nasal and vaginal ulcers, and Raynaud's phenomenon (less common).
2. **Musculoskeletal system** (MSK): generalized arthralgia with morning stiffness is very common. Myalgia is common. Frank arthritis may involve the small joints of the hands and wrists (usually symmetrical, polyarticular and non-erosive). Deformities are very rare but include Jaccoud's arthropathy (*Fig. 2.12.6*) which occurs due to ligament laxity.
3. **Renal system**: hypertension and haematuria may be present. Oedema, weight gain and hyperlipidaemia are common physical findings related to nephrotic syndrome or volume overload with renal failure. Nephritis is the leading cause of mortality in SLE patients in the first decade.
4. **Nervous system**: the central and peripheral nervous system should be assessed. Headache, seizures and aseptic meningitis are common.
5. **Cardiopulmonary**: pleuritis or pericarditis (*see above*). SLE patients have a roughly 2.7× risk of heart failure (due to atherosclerosis).
6. **GI system**: abdominal pain, nausea, vomiting and diarrhoea can occur in up to 50% of patients with SLE.
7. **Ocular**: Sjögren's syndrome and conjunctivitis are common in SLE; however, more serious manifestations such as optic neuritis may develop and can threaten blindness.

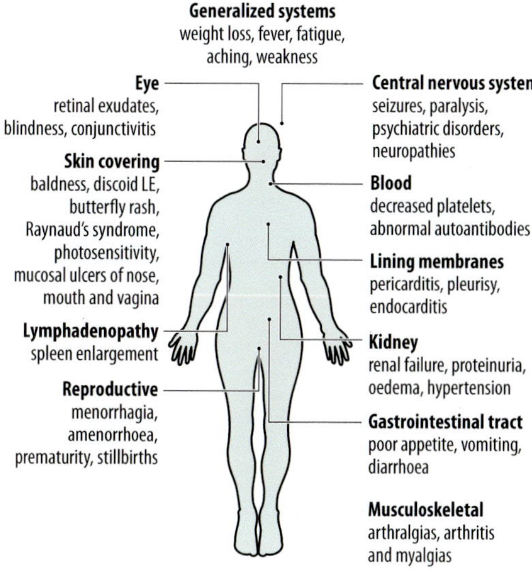

Fig. 2.12.2: SLE manifestations.

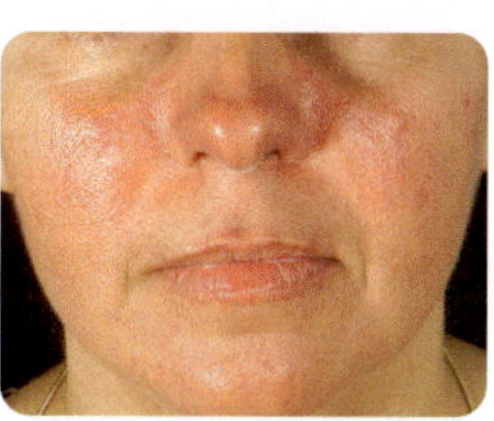

Fig. 2.12.3: Malar rash.

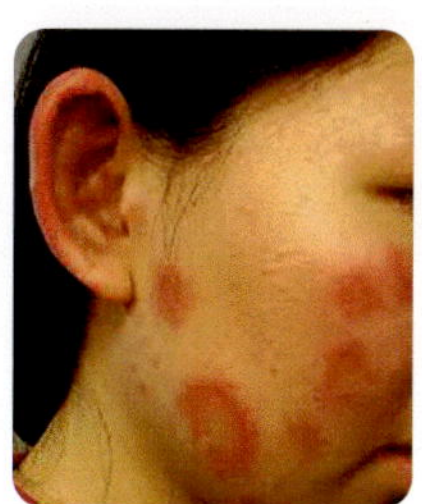

Fig. 2.12.4: Discoid rash.

Ix

- **Blood tests**:
  - FBC – anaemia, leucopenia, thrombocytopenia and rarely pancytopenia.
  - Activated prothrombin time – may be prolonged in patients with antiphospholipid antibodies.
  - ESR and CRP – elevated (non-specific).
  - Immunology – **ANA antibodies** (high sensitivity but low specificity), **anti-dsDNA** (highly specific), **anti-Smith antigen** (highly specific) positive, complement levels (C3, C4): ↓ levels show active disease and are usually associated with flares.
  - Urea and electrolytes – may be deranged if renal involvement.
- **Urinalysis**: haematuria, casts (red cell, granular, tubular or mixed) or proteinuria.
- **Chest X-ray**: all patients presenting with cardiopulmonary symptoms should have a chest X-ray performed for pleural effusion, infiltrates and cardiomegaly.
- **X-ray of affected joints**: periarticular osteopenia.
- **MRI**: in suspected CNS lupus.
- **ECG**: all patients presenting with cardiopulmonary symptoms should have an electrocardiogram (ECG). It may exclude other causes of chest pain.
- **Echocardiogram**: to investigate pericardial involvement.

DDx

- RA
- Antiphospholipid syndrome
- Systemic sclerosis
- Mixed connective tissue disease

Clinical facts: Complications of SLE

SLE patients are at increased risk of other serious conditions: **atherosclerosis**, **hypertension**, **dyslipidaemia**, **diabetes mellitus**, **osteoporosis**, **avascular necrosis**, **permanent neurological damage** and **lymphoma**.

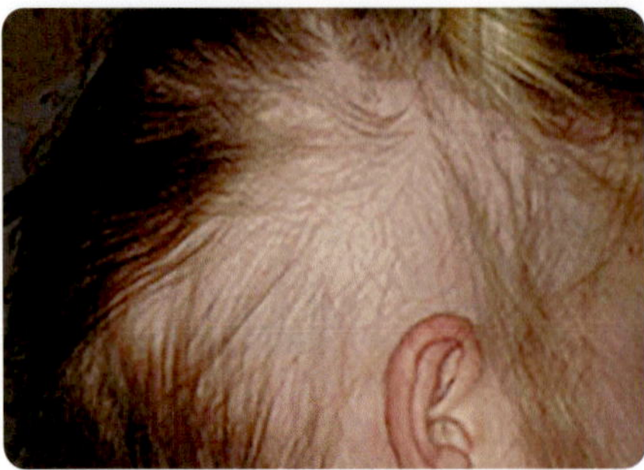

Fig. 2.12.5: Patient with alopecia.

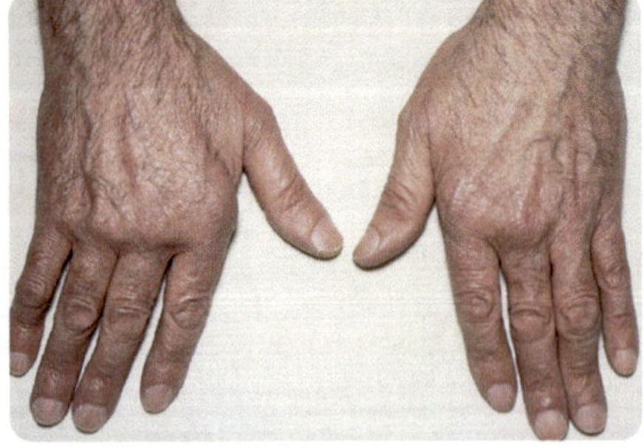

Fig. 2.12.6: Jaccoud's arthropathy.

Box 2.12.2: Antiphospholipid syndrome

Antiphospholipid syndrome (APS) may be associated with SLE but mostly exists as a primary disease. It is an important cause of recurrent arterial and venous thrombosis and miscarriages. It is associated with the presence of antiphospholipid antibodies.

Clinical features ('CLOT'):

Coagulation defects, Livedo reticularis, Obstetric (recurrent miscarriage), Thrombocytopenia.

Diagnosis (one clinical and one laboratory finding):

- Clinical – one episode of arterial and/or venous thrombosis, or morbidity in pregnancy
- Laboratory – anti-cardiolipin antibodies or lupus anticoagulant in plasma.

Management: low-dose aspirin, or warfarin if recurrent thromboses. Seek expert advice for pregnancy.

Management

Patient education

- **Advice about sun exposure** – patients with sun-induced rashes should use sunscreen regularly for about 6 months over the summer. Other patients with SLE should be aware that sun exposure may precipitate a flare.
- **Smoking cessation**.
- **Pregnancy and contraception** – pregnancy should be planned. Risk of problems with pregnancy is greatly reduced if disease is well controlled prior to conception. Drug therapy should be reviewed before pregnancy. Pills that contain oestrogen may exacerbate lupus disease or thrombosis and should be used with caution. In general, barrier methods or progesterone-only contraception are preferred.
- Infections should be avoided and treated promptly if appropriate.

Monitoring disease activity

- Anti-dsDNA antibody titres.
- Complement system: C3↓ C4↓, and C3d and C4d↑ suggests increased activity.
- ESR
- Others → BP, urinalysis for casts and protein, screening for organ damage, FBC, U & Es, LFTs, CRP (usually normal).

Pharmacological management

- **NSAIDs** for arthritis.
- **Hydroxychloroquine** for all patients with SLE (unless contraindicated). Be wary of retinal toxicity.
- **Glucocorticoids**: systemic steroids are used for acute flares and severe disease. Intra-articular steroids can be used for joint problems.
- **Topical agents** including calcineurin inhibitors (e.g. tacrolimus ointment) can be used for dermatological manifestations.

- **Immunosuppressants**:
  - Cyclophosphamide is often used for patients with severe renal, cardiac or neurological involvement or associated systemic vasculitis / autoimmune thrombocytopenia
  - Azathioprine, methotrexate and mycophenolate are often used as steroid-sparing agents
  - Biological drugs, e.g. rituximab, belimumab and anifrolumab may be used in refractory cases.
- When stable, treat-to-target strategies should be used (glucocorticoid tapering first).

Self-assessment

An 18 year old female presents to her GP with symptoms of fatigue, muscle pain and a facial rash. On examination she is noted to be thin with malar skin changes. No other abnormality is found. You suspect SLE.

1. What are the possible characteristic facial rashes that occur in SLE?
2. Name three risk factors of SLE.
3. What autoantibodies are present in almost all patients with SLE? Which autoantibodies are most specific to SLE?
4. How can the disease activity of SLE be monitored?
5. What general advice would you give to this patient?

Answers to self-assessment questions are to be found on the Resources tab at www.scionpublishing.com/Rheum2.

2.13 Polymyositis and dermatomyositis

Polymyositis (PM) is a rare idiopathic **heterogeneous group of conditions** characterized by **inflammation** and **weakness** of **skeletal muscle (proximal > distal)**. It may also affect other parts of the body such as **joints**, the **oesophagus**, **lungs** and **heart**. When PM pathology extends to the **skin**, the condition is termed **dermatomyositis** (DM). DM may coexist with other connective tissue disorders such as SLE.

Pathophysiology

- The pathophysiology of PM and DM remains largely uncertain but both environmental and genetic factors are likely to play a part in the disease process (*Fig. 2.13.1*).

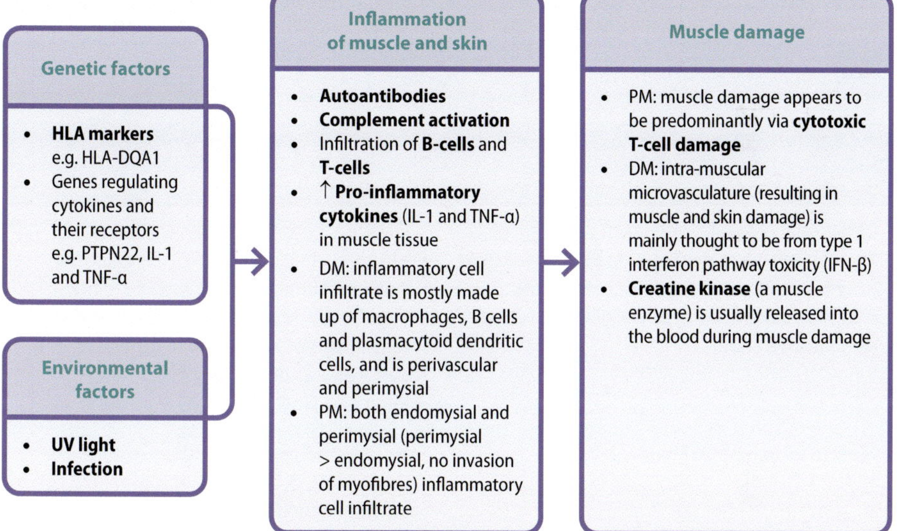

Genetic factors
HLA markers e.g. HLA-DQA1
Genes regulating cytokines and their receptors e.g. PTPN22, IL-1 and TNF-α
Environmental factors
UV light
Infection
Inflammation of muscle and skin
Autoantibodies
Complement activation
Infiltration of B-cells and T-cells
↑ Pro-inflammatory cytokines (IL-1 and TNF-α) in muscle tissue
DM: inflammatory cell infiltrate is mostly made up of macrophages, B cells and plasmacytoid dendritic cells, and is perivascular and perimysial
PM: both endomysial and perimysial (perimysial > endomysial, no invasion of myofibres) inflammatory cell infiltrate
Muscle damage
PM: muscle damage appears to be predominantly via cytotoxic T-cell damage
DM: intra-muscular microvasculature (resulting in muscle and skin damage) is mainly thought to be from type 1 interferon pathway toxicity (IFN-β)
Creatine kinase (a muscle enzyme) is usually released into the blood during muscle damage

Fig. 2.13.1: Overview of the pathophysiology of PM and DM.

Epidemiology and risk factors

- PM and DM are rare – the combined incidence is approximately 2–10 cases per million each year in the general population.
- There is an estimated prevalence of around 10 000 people in the UK.

Table 2.13.1: Risk factors for polymyositis and dermatomyositis	
Genetic predisposition	• There is an association between particular **HLA subtypes** such as HLA-DR3 and HLA-DR7 and increased risk of developing PM and DM.
Age	• DM has a **bimodal age distribution** with peaks at **5–15** and **45–60 yrs**. • PM is rare in childhood and occurs mainly in adults (peak **50–60 yrs**).
Female sex	• The overall female:male ratio is **2.5:1**.
Ethnicity	• PM and DM 3–4 × more common in **black people** than in Caucasians.
Malignancy	• DM may occur 2° to malignancy.
Environmental factors	• **UV light**: the rash in DM often develops in sun-exposed areas and some patients report photosensitivity. • **Infections**: viruses, bacteria and protozoa have been associated with DM.
Comorbidities	• Increased association with lupus, RA and Sjögren's syndrome.

Clinical features

PM	DM (presents with PM features and dermatological features)
Commonly presents with insidious, progressive and **symmetrical proximal muscle weakness** (weeks–months). The patient particularly experiences difficulties in walking up stairs or rising from a chair.	**Gottron's papules**: scaly, erythematous eruptions particularly over the extensor surfaces of the MCP, PIP and DIP joints (*Fig. 2.13.2*). Macular erythema (without scaly eruption) can occur in other extensor surfaces, e.g. of the elbows and knees, known as **Gottron's sign** (*Fig. 2.13.3*).
Muscle pain (approximately 1/3).	**Heliotrope rash**: violet discoloration of the eyelids, occasionally accompanied by periorbital oedema (*Fig. 2.13.4*).
Systemic features: fever, fatigue and weight loss (due to oesophageal dysmotility).	**Photosensitivity**
Aspiration pneumonia, **dysphagia**, **dysphonia** and **respiratory failure** (if there is involvement of the respiratory and pharyngeal muscles).	**Nail-fold erythema**
Pulmonary fibrosis (30%).	

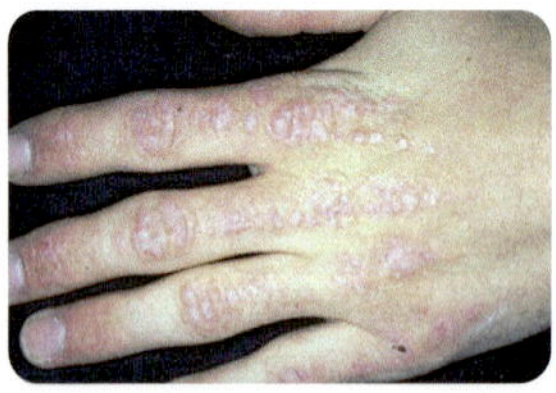

Fig. 2.13.2: Gottron's papules.

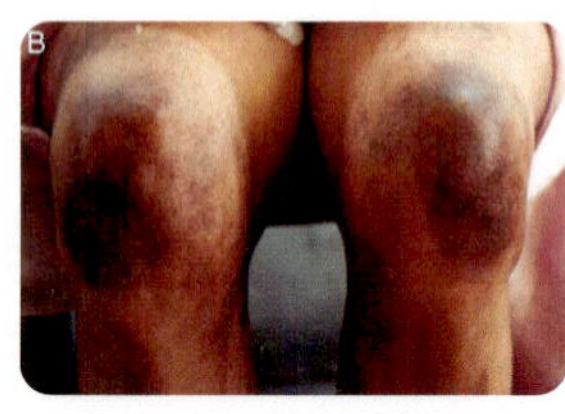

Fig. 2.13.3: Gottron's sign.

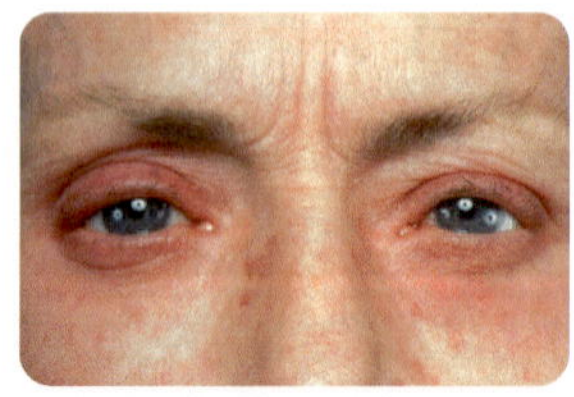

Fig. 2.13.4: Heliotrope rash.

Diagnosis and investigations

Hx

- See above for clinical presentation
- Risk factors, e.g. family history and recent infection
- Drug history – to exclude drug-induced myopathy

Ex

Polymyositis:

- **Proximal muscle weakness** and **atrophy** occur with comparative sparing of distal muscles.
- Difficulties in arising from sitting position due to involvement of pelvic girdle muscle.
- Forced flexion of the neck is weak.
- As muscular atrophy occurs, flexor plantar response and normal sensation are maintained.
- Muscles are **tender** on palpation.

Dermatomyositis (in addition to PM clinical features):

- **Gottron's sign and papules** – present in 60–80% of DM patients.
- **Heliotrope rash** – present in ≤50%.

For full details of the ACR/EULAR classification criteria, see *Box 2.13.1*.

Ix

Blood tests:

- **Creatine kinase** (CK) – can be up to 50 x higher than normal. It is rarely normal in active disease and the level is usually a good indicator of disease activity.
- Other enzymes are ↑ – aldolase, serum glutamic-oxaloacetic transaminase (SGOT), serum glutamic-pyruvic transaminase (SGPT), and lactate dehydrogenase (LDH).
- Myositis-specific antibody (MSA) and myositis-associated autoantibodies (MAA) may also be useful for diagnosis.
- **ESR**, **plasma viscosity** and **CRP** may be raised.
- Autoantibodies:
  - A positive **ANA** finding is found in approximately 60% of patients.
  - **Anti-Mi-2 antibodies** are specific for DM, but found in only 25% of patients.
  - **Anti-Jo-1 antibodies** are more common in patients with PM than in patients with DM. They are associated with interstitial lung disease, Raynaud's phenomenon and arthritis.

MRI: may show areas of inflammation, oedema, fasciitis in the muscle or fibre necrosis, and can be useful for monitoring disease activity.

Electromyography (EMG): abnormal but can be normal in up to 15% of patients with DM.

Muscle biopsy: confirms diagnosis. Shows evidence of myositis.

DDx

- Drug-induced myopathy (e.g. statins)
- Mixed connective tissue disease
- Hereditary neuromuscular diseases
- SLE

OSCE tips: Malignancy in DM

DM may occur 2° to a malignancy:

- Ask about **non-specific features of malignancy**, e.g. weight loss and malaise
- Perform **systems review**
- Consider performing **whole body CT**, **GI tract imaging** and **mammography**

Box 2.13.1: ACR/EULAR classification criteria for inflammatory myopathy (2017)

Points are presented as follows: 'without muscle biopsy' are first, and points 'with biopsy' second. A score of ≥7.5 without biopsy, or ≥8.7 with biopsy, is needed for classification.

Criterion	Without biopsy	With biopsy
Age:		
between 18 and 40	+1.3	+1.5
>40	+2.1	+2.2
Muscle weakness:		
Objective and symmetrical weakness of upper limb	+0.7	+0.7
Objective and symmetrical weakness of lower limb	+0.8	+0.5
Neck flexors weakness > extensors	+1.9	+1.6
Legs proximal weakness > distal	+0.9	+1.2
Skin signs:		
Heliotrope rash	+3.1	+3.2
Gottron's papules	+2.1	+2.7
Gottron's sign	+3.3	+3.7
Dysphagia or oesophageal dysmotility	+0.7	+0.6
Bloods:		
Anti-Jo-1 (+)	+3.9	+3.8
Elevated CK/LDH/(AST, ASAT, SGOT)/(ALAT, ALT, SGPT)	+1.3	+1.4
Biopsy:		
Endomysial infiltration surrounding (not invading) myofibres		+1.7
Perimysial infiltration		+1.2
Perifascicular atrophy		+1.9
Rimmed vacuoles		+3.1

Subgroups can be identified through clinical presentation

Management

Non-pharmacological

- **Sun-blocking agents** should be used for DM.
- Encourage **physical activity** in order to maintain muscular strength. Involvement of a **physiotherapist** and **occupational therapist** may be beneficial. A bone health assessment should be performed.
- Evaluation of swallowing may be required. **Speech and language therapist** may help with difficulties of swallowing.
- Monitor CK levels.
- Screen thoroughly for malignancy in DM.
- Screen thoroughly for interstitial lung disease and cardiovascular involvement.

Pharmacological

- Start high-dose **prednisolone**: 40–60 mg/24 hours. The dose should be gradually reduced according to the clinical response of CK levels. IV methylprednisolone can be considered as an alternative.
- **DMARDs** and **steroid-sparing drugs** can be used in early resistant cases, e.g. azathioprine, tacrolimus, methotrexate, ciclosporin and rituximab.
- **Intravenous immunoglobulins** may help in some patients.
- **Hydroxychloroquine** and **tacrolimus** may help with skin disease.
- **Rituximab** can also be considered with persistent skin disease.

Self-assessment

A 47 year old woman presents with a 5 week history of progressive weakness in her thighs and upper arms. She has difficulty getting out of a chair unaided and complains of fatigue and breathlessness. On examination, proximal muscle strength is symmetrically reduced but distal muscle strength is normal. Chest examination reveals fine bilateral basal crepitations. You suspect polymyositis.

1. What skin features help to distinguish dermatomyositis from polymyositis?
2. What blood tests would you perform on this patient and why?
3. What further definitive tests can be performed?
4. What is the first-line pharmacological treatment for this patient? What other options can be used in resistant cases?
5. How would you measure the clinical response to treatment?

Answers to self-assessment questions are to be found on the Resources tab at www.scionpublishing.com/Rheum2.

2.14 Sjögren's syndrome

Sjögren's syndrome (SS) is an **autoimmune disorder** of unknown cause characterized by **inflammation** of the **salivary**, **lacrimal** and other **exocrine glands.** The disease is referred to as **primary** if it develops in isolation, and **secondary** if it occurs with other autoimmune diseases, usually **RA**, **SLE** or **scleroderma**.

Pathophysiology

- **Environmental** or **endogenous antigens** trigger an **immune-induced inflammatory** response in **susceptible individuals**.
- **Hypergammaglobulinaemia** and **serum autoantibodies** (towards RF, Ro and La) lead to B-cell hyperactivity.
- The close relationship between **primary SS** and **SLE** has led to the suggestion that primary SS is likely to share similar features to the pathogenesis of SLE.
- There is particular **focal lymphocytic infiltration** (activated T cells in exocrine glands) and **fibrosis** of the **lacrimal** and **salivary glands** (mainly B cells) producing the main symptoms of **xerophthalmia** (**dry eyes**), **xerostomia** (decreased saliva production) and enlargement of the **parotid glands**.
- **Ductal** and **acinar epithelial cells** play a role in stimulating autoimmune injury by acquiring the ability to signal lymphocyte activation, producing pro-inflammatory cytokines and chemokines, and displaying immunoregulatory molecules (ICAM + CD40).
- Other organs may also be involved, but this occurs less commonly.

Epidemiology and risk factors

- The prevalence of Sjögren's syndrome in the UK is approximately 1.2%.

Table 2.14.1: Risk factors for Sjögren's syndrome

Female	Female:male **ratio 9:1**.
SLE	Significant overlap with SS.
RA	Significant overlap with SS.
Scleroderma	Significant overlap with SS.
HLA markers	HLA class II markers -A1, -B8, or -DR3/DQ2 haplotype are linked with susceptibility to SS.
Age	Peaks at 40s–60s and after menopause. Age at diagnosis may be years after symptom onset.
Family history	Confers susceptibility.

Clinical features ('D factor')

- **Keratoconjunctivitis sicca** (**d**ry eyes).
- **Xerostomia** (**dry mouth**).
- **Parotid swelling** (*Fig. 2.14.1*).

} Most common specific features

- **Vaginal dryness** and **dyspareunia**, **dry cough** and **dysphagia** (other glands).

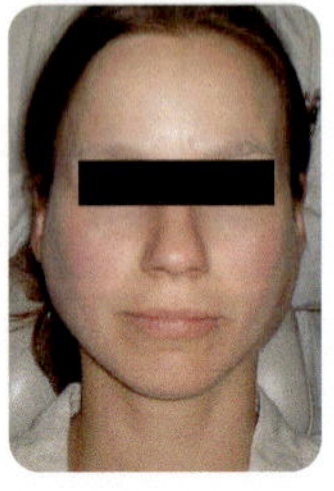

Fig. 2.14.1: Bilateral parotid swelling in SS.

- **Systemic features**: polyarthritis, arthralgia (60%), Raynaud's (37%), lymphadenopathy, vasculitis (9%), lung (14%), kidney (9%) and liver (6%) involvement, peripheral neuropathy, myositis and fatigue (25%).
- It is associated with other autoimmune diseases, e.g. SLE, and there is an increased risk of **non-Hodgkin's B-cell lymphoma**.

Diagnosis and investigations

Hx

- **Clinical presentation**: fatigue, dry eyes and dry mouth are all common.
- **Key risk factors**: female gender, SLE, systemic sclerosis, RA, HLA type II, age (40s–60s) and post-menopause.

Ex

- **Eyes**: dilatation of the conjunctival vessels may be present. Look for corneal lesions and gently pull down the lower eyelid to assess the tear pool. Blepharitis may be present.
- **Mouth**: may look dry and a wooden tongue depressor may stick to the tongue. There may be evidence of oral candidiasis and dental caries. Submandibular glands may be enlarged but bilateral enlargement of the parotid glands is more obvious.
- **Features of other autoimmune disorders**: most commonly RA, SLE and scleroderma.

Ix

- **Schirmer's test** (*Fig. 2.14.2*): quantitatively measures tears. A filter paper is placed in the lower conjunctival sac. The test is positive if less than 5 mm of paper is wetted after 5 minutes.
- **Blood tests**:
  - Antibodies to the ribonucleoproteins 60 kD **Ro** (SS-A) and **La** (SS-B) are found in up to 90% of patients with SS.
  - Raised ESR, hypergammaglobulinaemia, low C4.
  - Positive ANA and RF.
- **Salivary gland or lip biopsy**: shows lymphocyte infiltration and destruction of tissue.
- **Lissamine green test and rose Bengal staining**: may show keratitis.
- **Salivary gland scintigraphy**: decreased salivary gland function.
- **Parotid sialography**: gross distortion of the normal pattern of parotid ductules together with significant retention of contrast material.

DDx

- SLE
- RA
- Scleroderma
- Salivary gland tumours
- Sarcoidosis

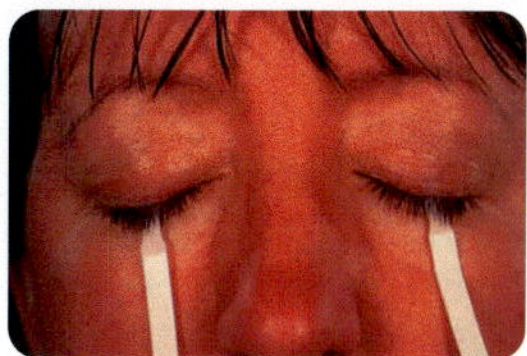

Fig. 2.14.2: Schirmer's test.

Rapid diagnosis: ACR/EULAR Consensus Group classification criteria (2016)	
Requires at least one symptom of ocular/oral dryness and does not have: active hep. C infection, history of head and neck radiation treatment, AIDS, sarcoidosis, amyloidosis, GvH, or IgG4-related disease. A score of ≥4 is required to classify as primary Sjögren's syndrome.	**Score**
1. **Objective ocular signs:** rose Bengal testing, lissamine green and fluorescein (≥5) or van Bijsterfeld (≥4)	**1**
2. **Schirmer's test** ≤5 mm/5 min in at least one eye	**1**
3. **Involvement of salivary gland by functional testing:** salivary scintigraphy, parotid sialography. Whole saliva flow rate ≤0.1 ml/min	**1**
4. **Anti-Ro (+) ± anti-La autoantibodies**	**3**
5. **Focal lymphocytic sialadenitis** on salivary gland biopsy and focus score ≥1	**3**

Management

- There is no specific treatment for SS but symptoms can be relieved by using topical treatments first and systemic therapies for active systemic disease.
- Baseline evaluation of gland function should be performed before treatment.

Dry eyes	• **Artificial tears** are first-line therapy. • **Ophthalmic ciclosporin drops / topical NSAIDs / corticosteroids** (maximum 2–4 weeks) can also be given. • **Spectacle eye shields** – a recommended adjunct to help maintain a humid environment. Also, patients should take regular breaks while reading. • **Humidifiers** – to alleviate loss of secretions by evaporation.
Dry mouth	• Patients should be encouraged to drink plenty to keep the mouth moist. • **Cholinergic drugs** to stimulate secretion of exocrine glands, e.g. **pilocarpine** and **cevimeline**. • **Salivary substitutes** for improving lubrication and hydration of oral tissues are used alone as first-line therapy.
Other features	• **Vaginal lubricants** may be required and infections such as vaginal candidiasis are more likely. • **Emollients** – may benefit dry skin. • **Hydroxychloroquine/NSAIDs** – may be useful in suppressing arthralgia and skin symptoms. • Glucocorticoids can be used for systemic disease; however, they should be tapered when possible, using synthetic immunosuppressive agents. • **B-cell targeted therapy (rituximab)** can be considered for severe refractory disease.

- The **EULAR Sjögren's syndrome disease activity index (ESSDAI) (2009)** was developed to assess systemic involvement in primary SS. Factors analysed to develop the index included **constitutional, lymphadenopathy and lymphoma, glandular, articular, cutaneous, pulmonary, renal, musculoskeletal** involvement, **PNS, CNS, haematological** and **biological**. The score calculated can be used to help direct systemic treatment options.

Self-assessment

A 35 year old woman presents with fatigue and a history of positive ANAs. She has had a recurrent sensation of sand in her eyes and dry mouth for over 3 months. You suspect Sjögren's syndrome.

1. What other clinical features may they have?
2. Which malignancy is linked to this condition?
3. What autoantibodies are specific to SS?
4. What investigation would you perform specifically for dry eyes?
5. Outline an appropriate management plan for this patient's symptoms.

Answers to self-assessment questions are to be found on the Resources tab at www.scionpublishing.com/Rheum2.

2.15 Scleroderma

Scleroderma, which is Greek for 'hard skin', is an **autoimmune** connective tissue disorder that affects the skin and other organs. There are two main types: **localized** and **systemic sclerosis (SSc)**. Localized scleroderma is more common in children and is confined to the **skin** and **subcutaneous tissue**. Systemic scleroderma may be **limited** (limited cutaneous systemic scleroderma (lcSSc); also known as **CREST syndrome**), which accounts for 70% of cases. The remaining 30% of cases are **diffuse** (dcSSc).

Pathophysiology

- The exact pathophysiology is not fully known. However, three processes are agreed to be important in disease progression:
  1. Immune system activation (potential environmental trigger) and development of **autoimmunity and epigenetic change**. **ANA** is positive in 90% of patients with SSc.
     - SSc patients may also have autoantibodies against matrix metalloproteinases, angiotensin 2 receptors and other cell surface markers. These show receptor agonist activity and may have pathogenic roles.
     - There is the presence of perivascular infiltrate, mainly consisting of B and T cells.
  2. Up-regulation of certain cytokines (e.g. IL-1, -4, -6, IFN) and proliferation of fibroblasts and mesenchymal cells contributes to **overproduction and accumulation of collagen**, which leads to hardening of the tissue. Generally, this is a later sign of SSc and is triggered by inflammation and microvascular damage.
     - SSc patients usually have monocytes and fibroblasts which express a profibrotic phenotype. They also have higher levels of type 2 innate lymphoid cells and alternatively activated macrophages (involved with tissue remodelling).
     - The immune response and loss of tolerance is partly related to dendritic cells being activated by self-nucleic acids. The generation of autoantibodies may be related to altered B-cell homeostasis (elevated B-cell activating factor (BAFF) and a proliferation-inducing ligand (APRIL)) in SSc patients.
  3. Systemic sclerosis pathology and inflammation extends to **small blood vessels in multiple places**, which can result in serious comorbidities and mortality. Clinical manifestations of vasculopathy include **Raynaud's phenomenon** (see *OSCE tips*), digital ulcers, renal crisis (accompanied by hypertension), pulmonary hypertension, and abnormalities in nail fold capillaries.
     - Endothelial damage causes endothelial cells to become myofibroblasts, which results in fibroproliferative vasculopathy. This, along with hypertrophy of the vessel wall (luminal occlusion), causes a cycle of vasculopathy, eventually leading to small vessel destruction.

Epidemiology and risk factors

- The UK prevalence is 1:10 000.
- Although systemic sclerosis is rare, it has a high mortality rate.

Table 2.15.1: Risk factors for scleroderma	
Positive ANA	• 90% of patients with SSc are positive for **serum ANA**.
Family history	• First-degree family history of SSc increases the risk by 60%.
Gender	• Female:male ratio is **4:1**.
Age	• Localized scleroderma is more common in children and young adults. SSc is more common in older adults.
Environmental factors	• Triggering factors may include **cytomegalovirus** and **chemicals**. Exposure to **silica dust** is associated with **lcSSc**.

Clinical features

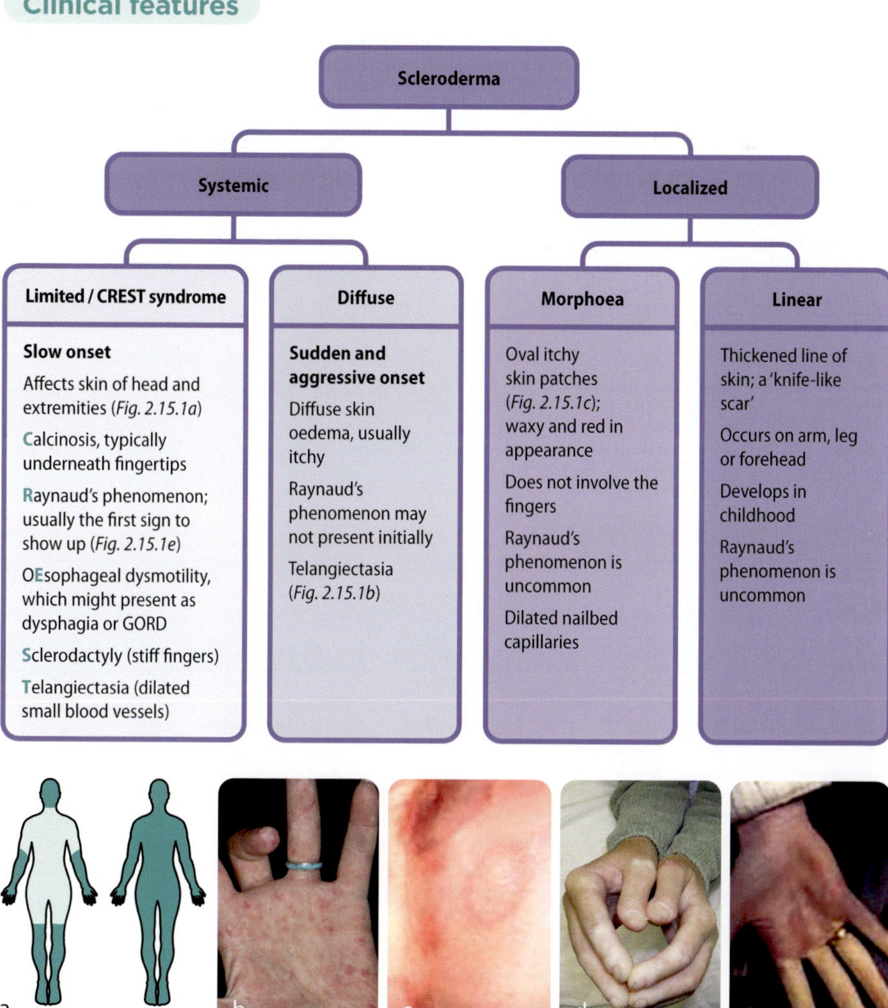

Scleroderma
Systemic
Localized
Limited / CREST syndrome
Slow onset
Affects skin of head and extremities (Fig. 2.15.1a)
Calcinosis, typically underneath fingertips
Raynaud's phenomenon; usually the first sign to show up (Fig. 2.15.1e)
OEsophageal dysmotility, which might present as dysphagia or GORD
Sclerodactyly (stiff fingers)
Telangiectasia (dilated small blood vessels)
Diffuse
Sudden and aggressive onset
Diffuse skin oedema, usually itchy
Raynaud's phenomenon may not present initially
Telangiectasia (Fig. 2.15.1b)
Morphoea
Oval itchy skin patches (Fig. 2.15.1c); waxy and red in appearance
Does not involve the fingers
Raynaud's phenomenon is uncommon
Dilated nailbed capillaries
Linear
Thickened line of skin; a 'knife-like scar'
Occurs on arm, leg or forehead
Develops in childhood
Raynaud's phenomenon is uncommon
a
limited
diffuse
b
c
d
e

Fig. 2.15.1: **(a)** Skin involvement distribution in SSc; **(b)** Telangiectasia (red spots); **(c)** Oval morphoea skin patch; **(d)** Prayer sign (unable to contact palmar surfaces together); **(e)** Raynaud's phenomenon (white/ischaemic colour stage).

- **Raynaud's phenomenon** is the first symptom in nearly all patients with SSc (especially lcSSc); the next symptoms usually appear within two years.
- **Skin thickness** is reliable diagnostic clinical sign; usually starts as **swelling and puffiness** of the skin (typically in the hands).
- SSc can affect internal organs:
    - Lung → **pulmonary hypertension** (15%), due to blood vessel damage, is a leading cause of mortality in patients with **lcSSc**. Overproduction of collagen can lead to **interstitial lung disease** (**dcSSc**) (65%).
    - Heart → **right heart failure** and **pericardial effusions**.
    - Kidney → **renal impairment**. Sclerodermal renal crisis occurs in about 15% of patients with dcSSc.
    - Gastrointestinal → **impaired peristaltic movement, bacterial overgrowth** and **GORD** (80%).
    - MSK → **synovitis (hands), calcifications of tendon sheaths** and **atrophy of skeletal muscle** (23%).

OSCE tips: Raynaud's phenomenon
WHITE → BLUE → RED!

- **Transient vasospasm** of the peripheral blood vessels (typically in the digits) leading to hypoxia. In extreme conditions it can cause **ischaemic gangrene** and **digital ulcers**.
- It is a common condition which affects 1–3% of population.
- **Stress** and **cold** are classic triggers of the phenomenon.
- Two types:
    - **Primary** (Raynaud's disease) which accounts for 90% of cases.
    - **Secondary** (10%) – usually due to connective tissue disorders such as SSc.
- Clinically diagnosed → **digits change colour** from **white** to **blue** to **red**.

Diagnosis and investigations

Hx

- Nature of **onset** and **duration** of signs and symptoms are key; dcSSc tends to have a faster progression than lcSSc.
- CREST syndrome → may present as gastro-oesophageal reflux disease (GORD, heartburn), dysphagia (liquids and solids), and weight loss.
- Risk factors including **family history** and **environmental factors**.

Ex

- Raynaud's phenomenon → initial sign for SSc.
- Hand swelling (earlier) and stiffness (later) due to thickened or hardened skin (worse in morning) with hair loss and pruritus → reduced range of movement (prayer sign; *Fig. 2.15.1d*).
- Note the extent of skin involvement.
- Subcutaneous calcinosis and telangiectasia.
- Foot swelling → prompt CVS examination (heart failure) and kidney function tests (renal impairment).
- Respiratory system examination → interstitial lung disease signs.

Ix

Blood tests:

- Haematology – usually normal.
  - ESR and WCC may be raised.
  - Anaemia of chronic disease.
- Immunology:
  - **ANA** – found in up to 90% of patients but lacks specificity.
  - **Anti-topoisomerase-1 (Scl 70)** antibody – associated with lung fibrosis and renal disease in both subsets of systemic sclerosis.
  - **Anti-centromere antibody (ACA)** – only in patients with CREST syndrome.
  - **Anti-RNA polymerase I and III antibody** – associated with diffuse scleroderma, especially with kidney involvement.
- Biochemistry:
  - Blood urea and creatinine – elevated in renal impairment.

Respiratory (lung involvement is major cause of mortality in SSc):

- Complete pulmonary function test – interstitial lung disease and pulmonary hypertension.
- Chest X-ray – interstitial lung disease, enlarged pulmonary arteries or enlarged right ventricle.
- High resolution CT – interstitial lung disease.

Cardiovascular system: echocardiogram shows raised pulmonary artery pressure and right ventricle dysfunction.

Gastrointestinal: barium swallow test (oesophageal dysmotility).

Nailfold capillaroscopy: abnormal capillary patterns (including dilatation, avascular areas and neo-angiogenesis) – suggestive of SSc.

Skin punch biopsy: may show features associated with lcSSc; however, this is rarely performed in practice as the histological features are not conclusive.

DDx

- Primary Raynaud's
- Other secondary causes of Raynaud's
- Other connective tissue disorders or mixed connective tissue disorders
- Scleromyxoedema
- Paraneoplastic syndromes

ACR/EULAR Consensus Group classification criteria for SSc (2013)

A score of ≥9 is required to classify as SSc

- Skin thickening on both hands from proximal to metacarpophalangeal joint (+9)
- Skin thickening of the finger: puffy fingers (+2), sclerodactyly of fingers (+4)
- Fingertip lesions: digital tip ulcer (+2), fingertip pitting scars (+3)
- Telangiectasia (+2)
- Abnormal nailfold capillaries (+2)
- PAH/ILD (+2)
- Raynaud's phenomenon (+3)
- Anti-centromere / anti-topoisomerase-1 (positive) (+3)
- Anti-RNA polymerase III (positive) (+3)

Management

Specific management is formulated dependent on the organ involved:

Skin	Skin hygiene and use of emollients for dry skin.
	Mycophenolate mofetil (MMF) first-line in dcSSc, with methotrexate as an alternative. Antihistamines may be useful for pruritus.
Vascular	Avoiding triggering factors for Raynaud's phenomenon.
	For Raynaud's use one of the following vasodilators: 1. **Calcium channel blockers (oral nifedipine)** 2. **Phosphodiesterase type 5 (PDE5) inhibitors,** e.g. sildenafil, tadalafil – also improves healing of digital ulcers. **Prostanoids (IV iloprost) for severe cases – this may also help heal digital ulcers.**
Gastrointestinal (potentially life-threatening)	Avoid eating 2–3 hours before bedtime and avoid caffeine.
	PPI inhibitors or **H_2-receptor agonists** for exacerbated conditions.
	Prokinetic drugs such as metoclopramide may be used for gut motility symptoms.
	Antibiotics for signs of GI infection (diarrhoea, unintentional weight loss and malabsorption).
Renal disease (potentially life-threatening)	An angiotensin-converting enzyme (**ACE**) **inhibitor / angiotensin receptor blocker (ARB)** for patients at risk of renal crisis.
	Renal transplantation may be considered if there is no significant renal recovery.

Cardiac (potentially life-threatening)	Oral prednisolone + close monitoring of blood pressure (cardiac tamponade) for patients with pericardial effusion.
	Immunosuppression and MMF for heart involvement with cardiac inflammation.
	Patients with cardiac tamponade require urgent medical care.
Pulmonary hypertension (potentially life-threatening)	An endothelin-receptor antagonist (ERA), PDE5 inhibitor or prostacyclin agonists.
Respiratory (potentially life-threatening)	**MMF** for patients with interstitial lung disease. Consider adding rituximab for progressive disease.
	Nintedanib is recommended for progressive pulmonary fibrosis.
	Haematopoietic stem cell transplantation may also be considered for patients at risk of organ failure, because it stabilizes lung function.
Cancer screening (>65 years)	Baseline screening (breast exam, lymphoreticular exam, FIT testing, endoscopy) recommended if there is a clinical phenotype for paraneoplastic syndrome.
	Chest, abdomen, pelvis CT may be considered by case.
	Follow-ups should be considered if there is clinical suspicion or risk factors (e.g. treated with high dose cyclophosphamide).

Self-assessment

A 39 year old woman complains of distal finger pain and tightening. She also has a history of Raynaud's for the past 4 years.

1. What clinical feature is illustrated in the patient's finger (*Fig. 2.15.2*)?
2. What is the most likely diagnosis?
3. What other signs would you look for during examination?
4. Which serum autoantibodies is she mostly likely to be positive for?

The patient revisits you after 6 months complaining of difficulty breathing.

5. What is the most likely underlying cause of her symptoms and what further investigations will you perform?

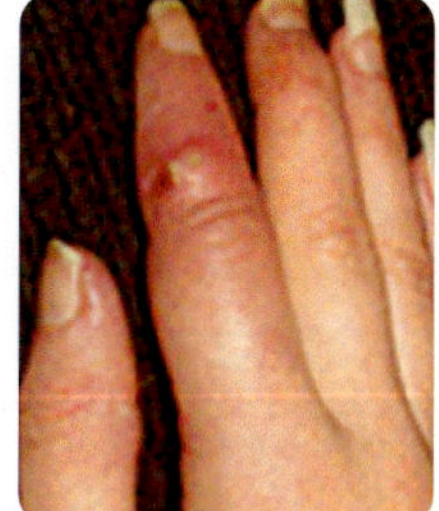

Fig. 2.15.2: Skin changes affecting the hand.

Answers to self-assessment questions are to be found on the Resources tab at www.scionpublishing.com/Rheum2.

2.16 Fibromyalgia

Fibromyalgia is a syndrome of **chronic pain** and the presence of **hyperalgesic points** at specific anatomical sites, as well as a range of other **physical** and **psychological symptoms** with **no identifiable organic cause**. This may overlap with other disorders where pain and fatigue are predominant symptoms, such as myalgic encephalomyelitis / chronic fatigue syndrome (ME/CFS).

Pathophysiology

- The cause of fibromyalgia is poorly understood but **abnormal central** and **peripheral pain processing** is thought to be responsible for **reduced pain threshold**, **hyperalgesia** (amplification of pain) and **allodynia** (pain produced by a non-noxious stimulus).
- This may be due to central pain sensitization and the loss of endogenous pain inhibitory mechanisms. There are also psychological elements (both emotional and cognitive) that play a part in pain perception with fibromyalgia patients.
- Some alterations in gene expression affecting metabolism and pain and stress pathways are seen in fibromyalgia patients and patients with other pain syndromes. This has led to fibromyalgia being considered part of the 'chronic overlapping pain syndromes' group.

Epidemiology and risk factors

- The prevalence of fibromyalgia in the general population is approximately 5.4%, but it is a condition that is underdiagnosed.
- The incidence of fibromyalgia in primary care in the UK is approximately 14 700 new cases per year.
- There are recognized risk factors for fibromyalgia but they only contribute approximately 5–10% to disease development (*Table 2.16.1*).

Table 2.16.1: Risk factors for fibromyalgia

Gender	• **10** × more common in **women** than men.
Age	• More common in individuals **aged 20–50**.
Physical trauma	• For example **whiplash type injuries** to the **neck** and **trunk**.
Psychological trauma	• **Stress, anxiety** and **depression**.
Viral infections	• May occur as a **post-viral syndrome**.
Family history	• There tends to be a familial increase in risk for fibromyalgia, and this may be due to some of the gene alterations seen in fibromyalgia.
Comorbidities	• RA, SLE, AS and OA all increase the risk of fibromyalgia.

Clinical features

'Fibro':

F	**Fatigue** (chronic) and **F**unctional impairment
I	**Insomnia** (and other sleep disturbances), **Irritability**, **Irritable bowel** and **Irritable bladder**
B	'Blues' – **anxiety** and **depression** (mood disorders experienced at some point by 80%)
R	**R**igidity – **muscle** and **morning joint stiffness**
O	'**O**w' – **pain** (widespread, chronic and functionally limiting) and others – **tender points** (*Fig. 2.16.1*), **paraesthesia**, **temperature changes**, **migraine**, **feeling of swollen joints**, **panic attacks**, **memory lapses** and **concentration deficit**

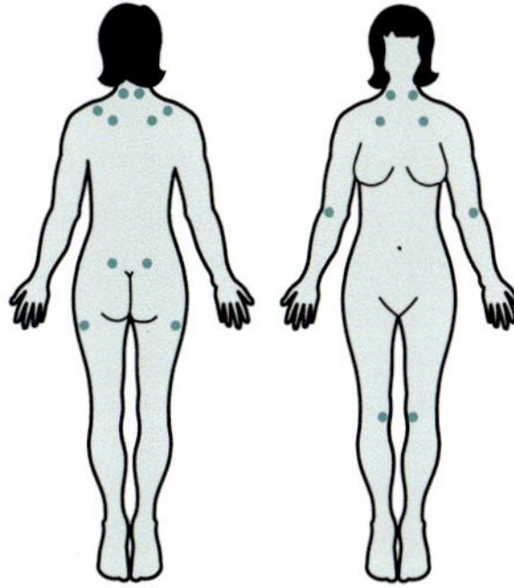

Fig. 2.16.1: Distribution of hyperalgesic tender points.

Diagnosis and investigations

Hx

- See above for symptoms and risk factors.
- A full **social**, **personal**, **family** and **psychological history** should be taken to reveal any past **physical trauma** or **psychological disturbance**.

Ex

- **Widespread pain**, above and below the waist as well as the axial skeletal system, for at least **3 months**.
- The presence of **11/18 tender points** shown in *Fig. 2.16.1*.
- **Digital palpation** using the thumb to assess tender points. The pressure applied should be just enough to blanch the examiner's thumbnail. In the absence of fibromyalgia, the palpation would not be enough to cause pain.
- **Systemic examination**: no abnormalities detected.

Ix

- **Blood tests** → normal
  - Haematology
  - Biochemistry
  - Immunology
- **Imaging** → normal

DDx

- ME/CFS
- Hypothyroidism
- Polymyalgia rheumatica
- Polymyositis

Yellow flags: Psychosocial risk factors for developing persisting chronic pain and long-term disability

- Belief that pain and activity are harmful
- Demonstration of sickness behaviour, e.g. prolonged rest
- Withdrawal from society
- Emotional problems – low mood, anxiety and stress
- Problems or dissatisfaction at work
- Problems with claims for compensation or time off work
- Overprotective family or lack of social support
- Inappropriate expectations of treatment

ACR Diagnostic Criteria 2010 (2016 proposals for modification)

1. **Widespread Pain Index (WPI) (range = 0–19)**
   Tally the number of areas in which the patient has had pain over the past week. In how many areas has the patient had pain? Score will be between 0 and 19.
   - Upper region: jaw, shoulder girdle, upper arm, lower arm (check left and right separately) (max. points = 8)
   - Lower region: hip (buttock, trochanter), upper leg, lower leg (check left and right separately) (max. points = 6)
   - Axial region: neck, upper back, lower back, chest, abdomen. (max. points = 5)
2. **Symptom Severity Scale (SSS) (range = 0–12)**
   Score 0–3 for each: fatigue, waking up unrefreshed, and cognitive symptoms over the past week.
   Score 0–1 for each: headaches, pain in lower abdomen, and depression having occurred in the last 6 months.
3. **Generalized pain in ≥4 regions for at least 3 months** (excluding jaw, chest, and abdominal pain).

Diagnosis can be made if (a) WPI ≥7, SSS ≥5 and criterion 3 is met, or (b) WPI 4–6, SSS ≥9 and criterion 3 is met.

Management (based on EULAR recommendations, 2016)

General points

- Pain and function should be assessed in a psychosocial context.
- Access to a **multidisciplinary team** with treatments taking into account the **patient's needs** including **pain intensity**, **function**, **depression**, **fatigue** and **sleep disturbance**.
- Potential pain generators (arthritis, bursitis or neuropathies) should be identified, as well as triggering conditions which need to be treated.
- Patient education and information should always be provided.

Non-pharmacological	
Heated pool treatment	Can improve pain and function with or without exercise.
Exercise programmes	Individually tailored exercise programmes which include **aerobic training** and **muscle strengthening**.
Cognitive behavioural therapy (CBT)	A form of **psychotherapy** that is based on scientific principles that help people change the way they think, feel and behave.
Meditation and mindfulness	Can be helpful in improving sleep and pain perception.
Others	**Relaxation**, **rehabilitation**, **acupuncture** and **psychological support**.
Pharmacological	
Mild pain relief	**Paracetamol** and weak opioids such as **codeine** can be considered (SIGN 2019).
Antidepressants (serotonin–noradrenaline reuptake inhibitors and tricyclic)	Reduce pain, e.g. **duloxetine** and **amitriptyline**. Minor improvement to sleep and functional impairment.
Neurotransmitter modulators (pregabalin and gabapentin)	May reduce pain by up to 30% and slightly improve sleep and functional impairment. However, these should be used with caution as they may have addictive potential and have been reclassified as Class C schedule drugs (SIGN 2019).

Self-assessment

A 40 year old woman complains of muscle pain all over the body and lack of sleep. On examination, tender symmetrical spots are identified on multiple sites.

1. What is the most likely diagnosis?
2. What would you expect to see if routine blood tests are performed?
3. Name two non-pharmacological approaches which can be offered.
4. What pharmacological agents are most likely to be effective for this condition?

Answers to self-assessment questions are to be found on the Resources tab at www.scionpublishing.com/Rheum2.

2.17 Osteoporosis

Osteoporosis is a **progressive**, **systemic skeletal disorder** characterized by **low bone mass** and **micro-architectural deterioration** of **bone tissue**, with a resultant increase in **bone fragility** and susceptibility to **fracture**. Osteoporosis exists when **bone mineral density (BMD)** values are reduced by more than **2.5 standard deviations** below that observed in **young healthy adults**.

Pathophysiology

- The underlying cause of osteoporosis is excessive **bone resorption** by **osteoclast cells** at a rate that exceeds **bone formation** by **osteoblast cells**.
- This results in **decreased bone mass** and **incomplete bone remodelling**, leading to disordered **bone architecture**.
- **Oestrogen deficiency** as a result of **menopause** is the commonest cause of osteoporosis. It commonly affects trabecular bone, which has a much larger area than cortical bone.
- **Oestrogen deficiency** → ↑ production of **RANK ligand (RANK-L)** by **osteoblasts** → ↑ **osteoclast formation**, **function** and **survival** → ↑ **osteoclastic activity** → ↑ **bone resorption** → ↓ **osteoblast lifespan** → ↓ **BMD**.
- Individuals with **inherited low peak bone mass**, **impaired absorption / inadequate intake of calcium**, **long periods of inactivity (disability)**, and other coexisting **metabolic bone diseases** such as **hyperparathyroidism** (may be secondary to vit D deficiency) → ↑ risk of osteoporosis.
- Long-term use of **glucocorticoid therapy** ↓ **osteoblastic activity** → ↑ risk of osteoporosis.
- Smoking has toxic effects on osteoblasts and may also alter oestrogen pathways, resulting in an increased risk of osteoporosis.
- Based on the **pattern of bone loss** and **fracture**, osteoporosis can be classified (*Fig. 2.17.1*) as:

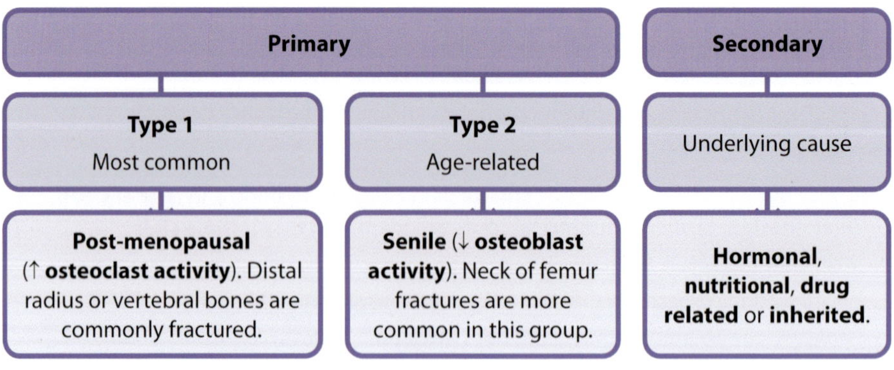

Primary
Secondary
Type 1
Most common
Type 2
Age-related
Underlying cause
Post-menopausal (↑ osteoclast activity). Distal radius or vertebral bones are commonly fractured.
Senile (↓ osteoblast activity). Neck of femur fractures are more common in this group.
Hormonal, nutritional, drug related or inherited.

Fig. 2.17.1: Classification of osteoporosis.

Epidemiology and risk factors

- It is estimated that over **2 million women have osteoporosis (in England and Wales)** (NICE CKS: *Osteoporosis – prevention of fragility fractures*, revised April 2023).
- The prevalence of osteoporosis in women is roughly 2% at 50 yrs and nearly 50% at 80 yrs.
- Risk factors include **female sex**, **family history** and '**SHATTERED**':

S	**Steroid use**, **Smoking**
H	**Hyperthyroidism**, **Hyperparathyroidism**, **Hypercalcinuria**
A	**Age** (>50), **Alcohol**
T	**Thin** (BMI <22)
T	**Testosterone deficiency**
E	**Early menopause**
R	**Renal, liver failure**
E	**Erosive bone disease**, e.g. RA or myeloma
D	**Deficiency of calcium and / or vitamin D, Diabetes, Drugs such as thyroid hormone, anticonvulsants, PPIs, aromatase inhibitors and thiazolidinediones**

Clinical features

- Usually **asymptomatic**.
- Clinical signs arise with fractures which commonly occur in the **spine** (*Fig. 2.17.2*), **hip** (*Fig. 2.17.3*) and **wrist** (*Fig. 2.17.4*):
  - **Back pain**, **reduced height**, **kyphosis** and **respiratory difficulty** (vertebral fracture).
  - **Painful**, **shortened** and **externally rotated hip** (hip fracture).
  - **Pain** and **deformity** (wrist / other fractures).

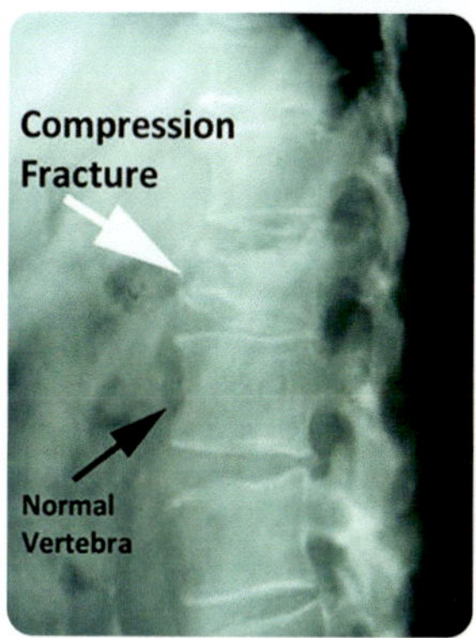

Fig. 2.17.2: Old osteoporotic compression fracture.

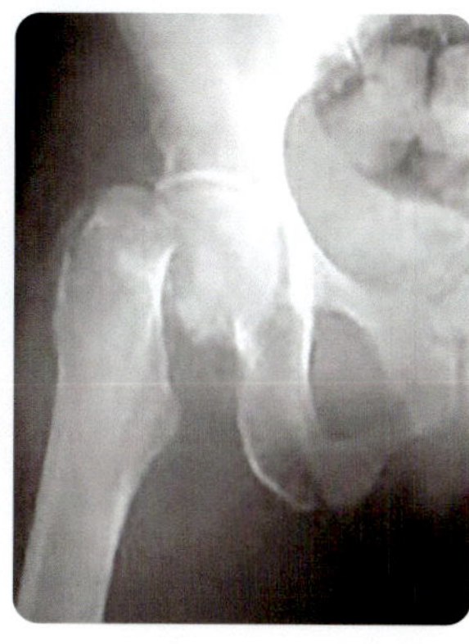

Fig. 2.17.3: Intra-capsular neck of femur fracture.

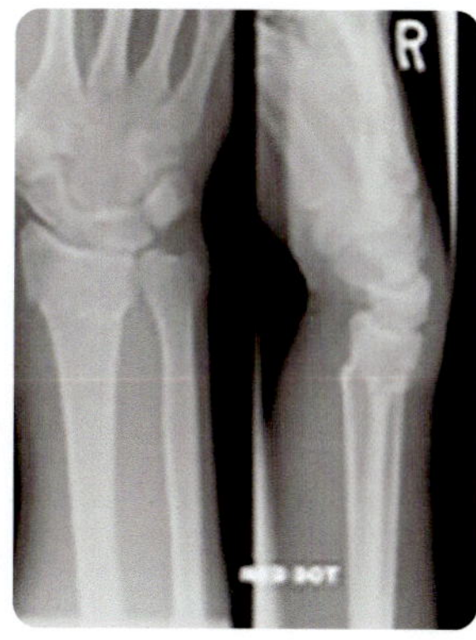

Fig. 2.17.4: Colles' wrist fracture.

Diagnosis and investigations

Hx

- Usually **asymptomatic** unless a fracture is present.
- Ask about **risk factors**, e.g. **steroid use**, **family history** and **menopause**.

Ex

- **Height loss** and **kyphosis** (vertebral fracture).
- **Painful**, **shortened** and **externally rotated hip** (hip fracture).
- **Pain** and **deformity** (other fractures).

Ix

Blood tests:

- **↑ Parathyroid hormone (PTH) levels → hyperparathyroidism**
- **Thyroid function tests (TFT) → ↑ T3, T4; ↓ TSH (hyperthyroidism)**
- **↑ Serum FSH, ↓ sex hormones, ↓ androgens → sex hormone deficiency / menopause**
- **↓ Vitamin D → vitamin D deficiency**
- **↑ ESR → inflammatory disease**, e.g. **RA** or **myeloma**
- **Bone biomarkers**, e.g. **calcium** and **alkaline phosphate** are usually normal

X-ray: to **confirm fracture** (if suspected); cannot determine if patient has osteoporosis but can predict if bones are **osteopenic**.

Dual-energy X-ray absorptiometry (DEXA) scan: works out the **BMD** of the patient in the **spine** and **hip**; two scores are calculated:

- **T-score** → diagnostic of osteoporosis; gives the number of **standard deviations** the **BMD** is from a **young healthy adult** (*Table 2.17.1*)
- **Z-score** → compares an individual's results to others of the **same age** and **gender**; **a Z-score of <−1.5** raises concern of factors other than ageing contributing to osteoporosis.

Fracture risk (FRAX): 10-year risk of hip / major osteoporotic fracture, estimated by incorporating BMD, age, gender and other clinical risk factors.

DDx

- Osteomalacia
- Paget's disease
- Hyperparathyroidism
- Multiple myeloma

Table 2.17.1: WHO osteoporosis criteria

T-score	Interpretation
>0	BMD better than reference population
0 to −1	No evidence of osteoporosis
−1 to −2.5	Osteopenia
−2.5 or below	Osteoporosis
−2.5 or below plus fracture	Established osteoporosis

Clinical facts: Osteoporosis

- Osteoporotic fractures cause significant **morbidity** and ↑ the likelihood of **mortality**.
- **Hip fractures** have the **highest morbidity** and **mortality**, with **20–30%** of patients dying within the **first year** of fracture.
- The **Fracture Risk Assessment Tool (FRAX)** can be used to predict fractures. This should be calculated for all men >75 and women >65 yrs. It can be calculated earlier if risk factors are present. A score of >10% should be followed by a DEXA scan.

Management

Non-pharmacological management

Smoking cessation and **reduction** in **alcohol** consumption, weight-bearing muscle **exercises**, **dietary** (adequate source of **calcium** and **vitamin D**), **physiotherapy**, assessment of home **safety** and reducing the risk of falls (especially in the elderly).

Pharmacological management

See *Table 2.17.2*.

Table 2.17.2: Pharmacological management of osteoporosis based on NOGG recommendations (2024)

Bisphosphonates	First-line. **Inhibit bone resorption** by **inhibiting osteoclasts**. Examples include **alendronate** (**first-line**), **risedronate** (men) and **zoledronate** (post hip fracture). Can be taken orally once a week (alendronate) or as once-yearly IV injections (zoledronate). **GI side-effects** are common with oral medication and patients are asked to sit or stand for at least 30 minutes to reduce side-effects of **oesophagitis**.
Denosumab	**Monoclonal antibodies** directed against **RANK-L**. Used as an alternative treatment to bisphosphonates. Given as **6-monthly injections**.
Teriparatide and abaloparatide	**Parathyroid hormone analogues**. **Intermittent** exposure to **parathyroid hormone** activates **osteoblasts** more than **osteoclasts** and thus stimulates **new bone formation**. Taken as a **once-daily injection** into the **thigh or abdomen**. Very **expensive**. Used in **high fracture risk cases**.

Table 2.17.2: Pharmacological management of osteoporosis based on NOGG recommendations (2024) *(continued)*	
Romosozumab	This is recommended for treating severe osteoporosis in post-menopausal women and used under specialist guidance. It is a monoclonal antibody that inhibits sclerostin and so increases bone formation.
HRT	Typically used in those with premature ovarian failure or early menopause. Helps reduce bone loss and increases osteoblast lifespan.
Other	**Raloxifene, tibolone** – these are less commonly used but can be trialled if bisphosphonates are not tolerated or in younger post-menopausal women.

Self-assessment

A 32 year old man being treated for sarcoidosis develops back pain 6 months after steroid treatment was commenced. The radiologist reports a vertebral crush fracture and suggests that the 'bones look osteopenic in nature'. A diagnosis of osteoporosis is later confirmed with a DEXA scan.

1. Name three other risk factors of osteoporosis.
2. How could this have been prevented?
3. What first-line treatment would you prescribe? Name the most common side-effects.

A 43 year old woman has been complaining of amenorrhoea and hot flushes. The patient is later diagnosed with early menopause. A routine DEXA scan is performed and T-scores of −2.2 and −1.3 are reported in the vertebrae and hip, respectively.

4. What do the T-scores reveal in this patient?
5. What tool can be used to evaluate fracture risk?
6. What lifestyle advice would you recommend to this lady?

Answers to self-assessment questions are to be found on the Resources tab at www.scionpublishing.com/Rheum2.

2.18 Paget's disease

Paget's disease is a common bone disease that is often seen as an incidental finding on routine X-rays. It is characterized by focal increases in bone remodelling, resulting in the **abnormal production of bone** which is **mechanically weak, more vascularized and expanded**. The most commonly affected bones include the **pelvis**, **spine**, **skull**, **femur** and **tibia**. Patients are usually asymptomatic; however, they can experience pain due to bone expansion.

Pathophysiology

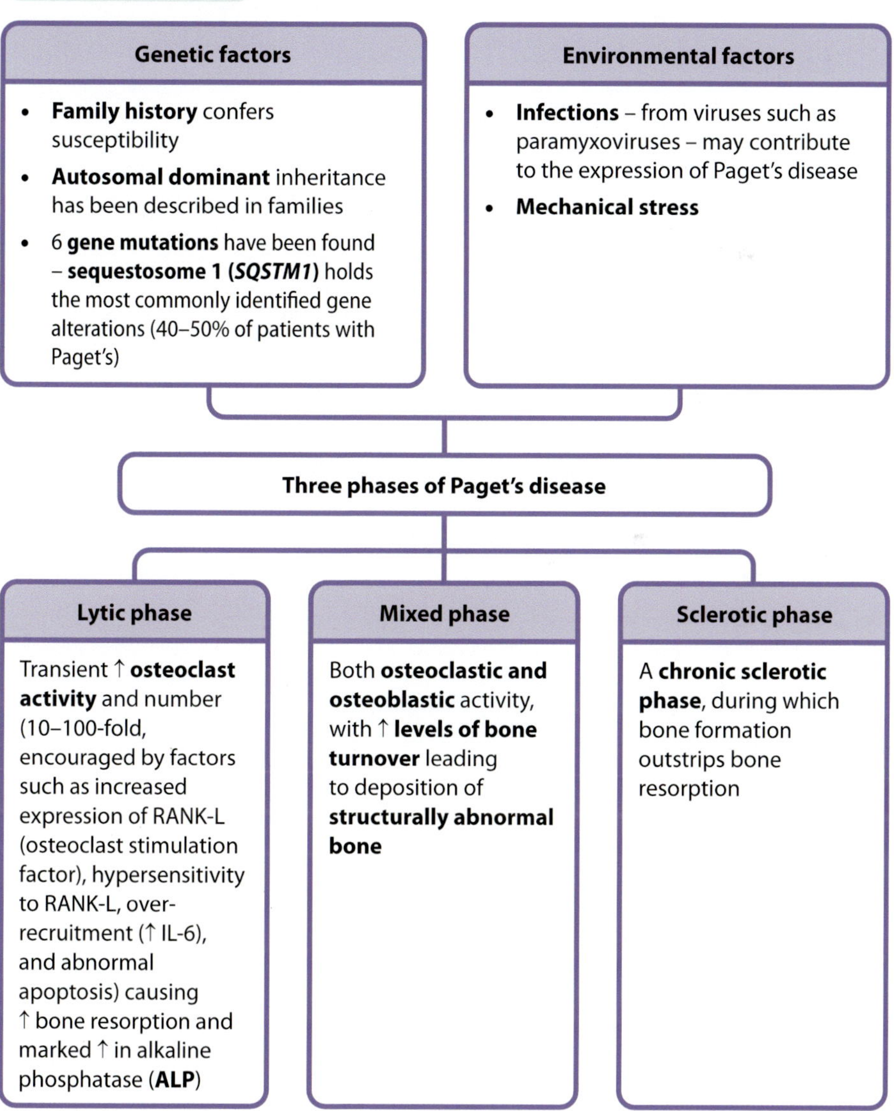

Genetic factors
• Family history confers susceptibility
• Autosomal dominant inheritance has been described in families
• 6 gene mutations have been found – sequestosome 1 (SQSTM1) holds the most commonly identified gene alterations (40–50% of patients with Paget's)
Environmental factors
• Infections – from viruses such as paramyxoviruses – may contribute to the expression of Paget's disease
• Mechanical stress
Three phases of Paget's disease
Lytic phase
Transient ↑ osteoclast activity and number (10–100-fold, encouraged by factors such as increased expression of RANK-L (osteoclast stimulation factor), hypersensitivity to RANK-L, over-recruitment (↑ IL-6), and abnormal apoptosis) causing ↑ bone resorption and marked ↑ in alkaline phosphatase (ALP)
Mixed phase
Both osteoclastic and osteoblastic activity, with ↑ levels of bone turnover leading to deposition of structurally abnormal bone
Sclerotic phase
A chronic sclerotic phase, during which bone formation outstrips bone resorption

Fig. 2.18.1: Outline of the pathophysiology of Paget's disease.

Epidemiology and risk factors

- The UK has a high prevalence of approximately 2% in Caucasians over the age of 55.
- The condition is very rare in Asians.

Table 2.18.1: Risk factors for Paget's disease	
Age	• The mean age of onset is approximately **55 years.**
Gender	• The male:female ratio is **2:1**.
Ethnicity	• Common in the UK but very rare in Asian countries.
Family history	• The relative risk can be **up to 7–10-fold** in **first-degree relatives** of patients with Paget's disease.

Clinical features

- Paget's disease is usually **asymptomatic** (**70–90%**) and therefore diagnosed on incidental abnormal X-ray or biochemical findings (↑ **ALP**).
- Complications depend on the site affected as well as the activity of the disease (*Table 2.18.2*).

Table 2.18.2: Typical complications of Paget's disease	
Bone pain	Most common
Bone deformity & enlargement	Typically the pelvis, lumbar spine, skull, femur and tibia (*Fig. 2.18.2*); may also be present as frontal bossing
↑ Temperature over affected bone	Due to hypervascularity
Muscle pain	Bone bowing may stretch muscles, causing pain
Pathological fractures	Due to mechanically weak bone; typically occurs in long bone
2° OA	Due to Paget's disease surrounding the joint
Hearing loss and tinnitus	Paget's disease affects the skull bones and may compress the vestibulocochlear nerve and cause other neurological symptoms

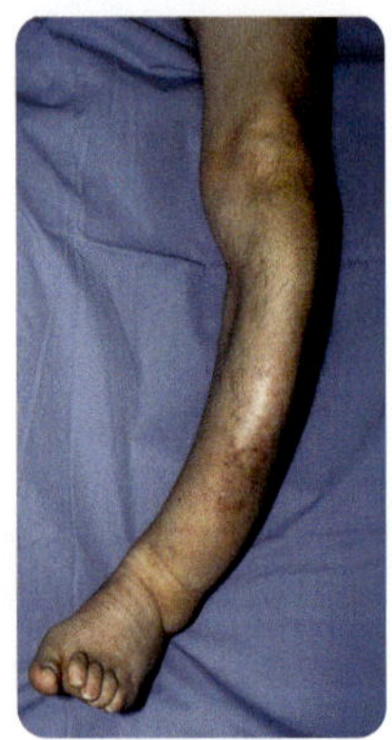

Fig. 2.18.2: Clinical bowing of the tibia in Paget's disease.

- **Less common complications**: spinal stenosis, nerve compression syndromes and cauda equina syndrome.
- **Rare complications**: hypercalcaemia, high output cardiac failure, paraplegia and osteosarcoma.

Diagnosis and investigations

Hx

- Usually **asymptomatic** but **bone pain**, **pathological fractures**, **deformities**, ↑ **local temperature** and **hearing loss** are all common.
- **Family history**.

Ex

- Look for head signs – ↑ **skull size**, **frontal bossing**, **deep-set eyes**, **large maxilla** with **prominent arches**.
- Look for other deformities such as **bowing** of **long bones** and **kyphosis**.
- Feel for **temperature** over affected bone.
- **Weber's** and **Rinne's test** – to elicit possible **sensorineural** hearing loss.
- Signs of other complications such as **OA** and **spinal cord compression**.

Ix

- **Blood tests**: ↑ **ALP**, **bone-specific ALP** (if known liver disease), phosphate and calcium are normal. **Procollagen type I *N*-terminal propeptide** (**PINP**) (bone formation marker) and serum **C-telopeptide** (**CTx**) (resorption markers) also reflect disease activity.
- **Urine tests**: **urinary *N*-telopeptide (NTx)** and **urinary hydroxyproline** are also markers of bone turnover.
- **X-ray** (*Figs 2.18.3* and *2.18.4*): **localized enlargement**, **patchy cortical thickening** with **sclerosis**, **osteolysis** and deformity, **advancing lytic lesion** in the long bones, vertebral deformities 'picture frame'/'ivory vertebra'.
- **MRI spine**: to exclude spinal stenosis, cord compression, or metastatic disease if suspected.
- **Radionuclide bone scan**: identify active skeletal lesions.

DDx

- Osteomalacia
- Osteoporosis
- Fibrous dysplasia
- Myeloma

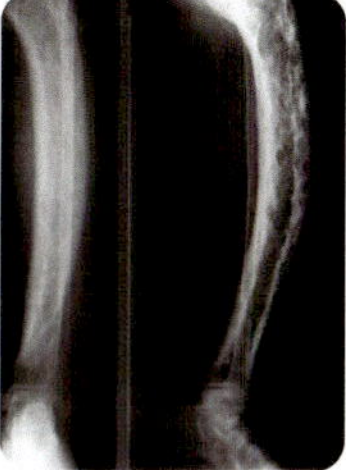

Fig. 2.18.3: X-ray showing the 'sabre tibia' in Paget's disease.

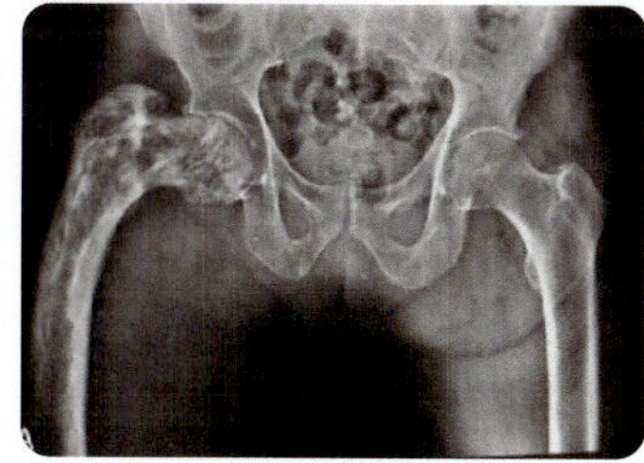

Fig. 2.18.4: X-ray of Paget's disease of the femur.

Management

Conservative management

- Observation, regular follow-up, patient education and preventive measures.
- Orthotic **devices**, **sticks** and **walkers** may be useful for Paget's disease of the legs.
- Adequate intake of **calcium** and **vitamin D**.

Pharmacological management

- Main indication is bone pain.
- **Bisphosphonates** to reduce bone turnover, e.g. oral risedronate or IV zoledronate.
- **Calcitonin** can be considered where bisphosphonates are not recommended.
- **Denosumab** may be efficacious; however, currently there is very little evidence supporting this.
- **NSAIDs** and **paracetamol** for pain relief.

Surgical management

- Bone deformity, osteoarthritis, pathological fractures and nerve compression may necessitate surgery.
- Surgical procedures include **fracture fixation** (pathological fracture), **joint replacement** (secondary OA), and **osteotomy** (deformity).

Self-assessment

A 50 year old man complains of constantly aching legs. Blood tests reveal an elevated level of serum ALP. Subsequent X-ray of the tibia shows a degree of tibial bowing. You suspect Paget's disease.

1. What other bone disorders can cause raised ALP?
2. What other bones are commonly affected in Paget's disease?
3. Apart from bone pain, name five other complications that can arise from Paget's disease.
4. How should this patient be managed pharmacologically?

Answers to self-assessment questions are to be found on the Resources tab at www.scionpublishing.com/Rheum2.

Chapter 3

Paediatric rheumatology conditions

3.1	Vitamin D deficiency	98
3.2	Juvenile idiopathic arthritis	103

3.1 Vitamin D deficiency

Vitamin D deficiency (also known as **hypovitaminosis D**) remains one of the most common vitamin deficiencies. There is an increasing reliance on dietary sources of vitamin D due to growing concerns about the effects of sun exposure. Vitamin D insufficiency is defined as a serum 25-hydroxyvitamin D level of <50 nmol/L and deficiency is defined as <30 nmol/L. It causes **inadequate mineralization of bone** and clinically manifests as **rickets** in children and **osteomalacia** in adults. It is associated with an increased mortality (particularly cardiovascular causes).

Pathophysiology

- Normal bone mineralization depends on adequate **calcium** and **phosphate** and this is maintained by vitamin D.
- **Vitamin D deficiency** is most commonly caused by inadequate ultraviolet B sunlight exposure for the formation of vitamin D_3 in skin.
- Vitamin D deficiency is commonly caused by failure of kidneys to **hydroxylate 25-hydroxyvitamin D (25-OHD)** to **1,25-dihydroxyvitamin D** in chronic kidney disease.
- Low levels of vitamin D impair calcium absorption in the intestines.
- This results in ↓ **mineralization of bone** via an ↑ **parathyroid hormone (PTH)** (secondary hyperparathyroidism) in response to ↓ **circulating levels of phosphate and calcium** (*Fig. 3.1.1*).
- Other causes of vitamin D deficiency are also shown in *Box 3.1.1*.

Box 3.1.1: Causes of vitamin D deficiency

- **Lack of sunlight** – especially those who routinely cover their face and hands (e.g. Muslim women) and those who are housebound (e.g. elderly individuals)
- **Renal disease** – due to impairment of C-1 hydroxylation of 25-OHD
- **GI malabsorption** – **coeliac disease**, **short bowel syndrome** and **cystic fibrosis**
- **Liver disease** – due to impaired C-25 hydroxylation of vitamin D
- **Drugs** – use of **anticonvulsants**, **rifampicin**, **cholestyramine**, **highly active antiretroviral treatment (HAART)**, or **glucocorticoids**
- **Genetic causes** – **hypophosphataemic rickets**, **type 1** (impaired C-1 hydroxylation) and **type 2 vitamin D resistance rickets** (target organ resistance).
- **Lack of dietary vitamin D sources** – particularly important for darker skin tones in low sunlight environments.
- **Hormone resistance due to receptor mutation or excess of hormones** – such as fibroblast growth factor 23 (FGF23), may also decrease vitamin D levels.

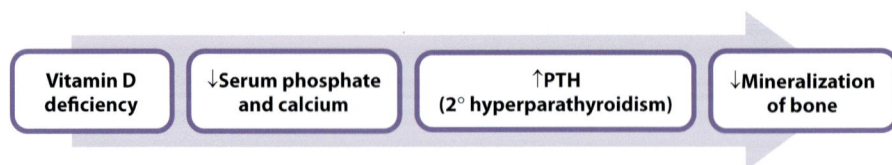

Vitamin D deficiency → **↓Serum phosphate and calcium** → **↑PTH (2° hyperparathyroidism)** → **↓Mineralization of bone**

Fig. 3.1.1: Overview of the pathophysiology of rickets / osteomalacia.

Epidemiology and risk factors

- Approximately 1 billion people worldwide have vitamin D deficiency.
- Vitamin D insufficiency (25(OH)D <50 nmol/L) affects 40% of the UK population, including 1 in 6 children and 1 in 5 adults.

Table 3.1.1: Risk factors for vitamin D deficiency

Dark skin	• **Afro-Caribbean, Middle Eastern** and **south Asians**.
Age	• **Children** and those **over 65 years**. May be related to behaviour and decreasing levels of 7-dehydrocholesterol.
Breastfeeding	• Infants who are exclusively breastfed beyond 6 months.
Obesity	• When BMI is >30, fat sequesters vitamin D, reducing bioavailability.
Routine covering of face and hands	• Common among **Muslim women** who wear veils.
Housebound	• Limited exposure to sunlight – particularly the **elderly**.
Sunscreen	• **Skin-concealing garments** or **strict sunscreen** use.
Pregnancy	• Multiple, short interval pregnancies.
Sex	• 1.3 female:1 male for insufficient levels of vitamin D (25(OH)D <50 nmol/L).
Environmental factors	• The ability of the skin to synthesize vitamin D may be affected by, for example, seasonal sunlight variations.

Clinical features

Rickets	Osteomalacia
***Infants*: growth retardation**, **hypotonia** and **apathy**.	**Bone pain** and **tenderness**.
***Once walking*: knock-kneed** (genu valgum; *Fig. 3.1.2*); **bow-legged** (genu varum; *Fig. 3.1.3*); **deformities of the metaphyseal–epiphyseal junction**; bone pain (typically pelvis and foot).	**Pathological fractures** (particularly femoral neck).
Hypocalcaemia (severe vitamin D deficiency typically accompanied by use of potent bisphosphonates or hypomagnesaemia) – paraesthesia, tetany, cramps, seizures.	**Proximal myopathy** causing proximal weakness, numbness (mouth, arms and legs) and possibly a waddling gait.

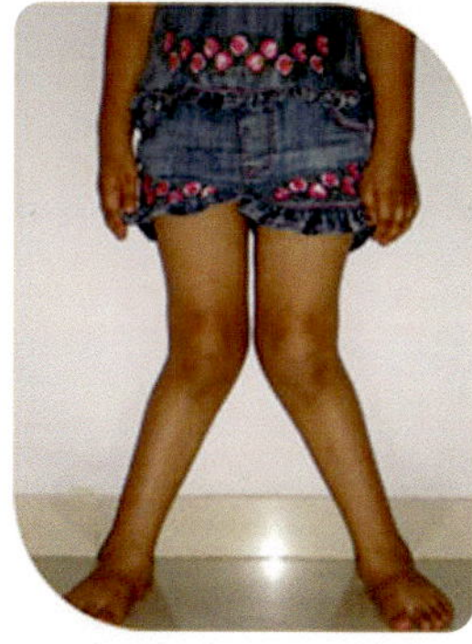

Fig. 3.1.2: Genu valgum.

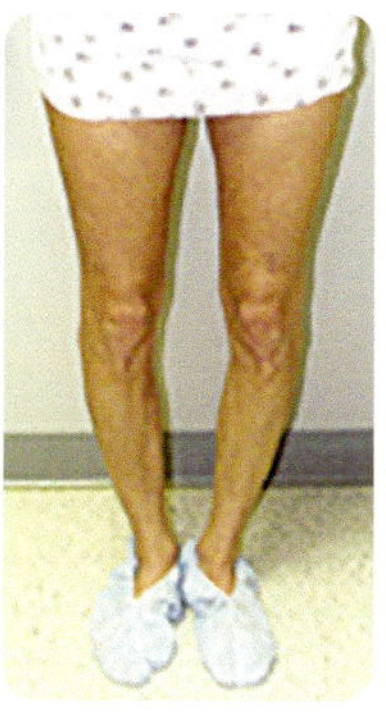

Fig. 3.1.3: Genu varum.

Diagnosis and investigation

Hx

- Explore **risk factors**.
- *Rickets* → failure to thrive, delayed achievement of motor milestones, fatigue and malaise, bowing of the legs, delayed tooth eruption and dental caries, chest deformity, and head sweating are all common.
- *Osteomalacia* → localized or generalized bone tenderness and muscle weakness. In severe cases there may be hand cramping / spasms.

Ex

- *Rickets* → bowing of the legs, widening of the bones, chest deformity and more (*Fig. 3.1.4*).
- *Osteomalacia* → bone tenderness (particularly in the back, pelvis and long bones of the leg), proximal muscle weakness and waddling gait, pathological fractures, and signs of hypocalcaemia.

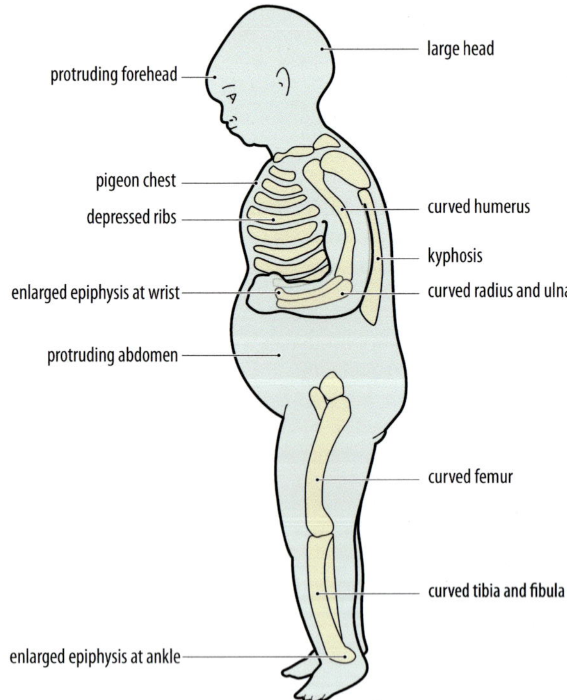

Fig. 3.1.4: Bone deformities in children with rickets.

Ix

Blood tests:

- ↓ **25 hydroxyvitamin D** (<30 nmol/L)
- →↓ $\mathbf{Ca^{2+}}$
- ↑ **PTH**
- ↓ **fasting phosphate**
- →↑ **ALP**

X-rays (of weight-bearing bones):

- *Osteomalacia:*
  - **Pseudofractures or Looser zones** are pathognomonic of osteomalacia. They are low-density bands extending from the cortex inwards in the shafts of long bones (*Fig. 3.1.5*)
  - **Coarse trabeculae**
  - **Osteopenia**
- *Rickets:*
  - **Metaphyseal cupping** and **flaring** – expansion of chondrocyte layer
  - **Epiphyseal irregularities**
  - **'Rachitic rosary'** – costochondral junctions
  - **Widening of the epiphyseal plates**

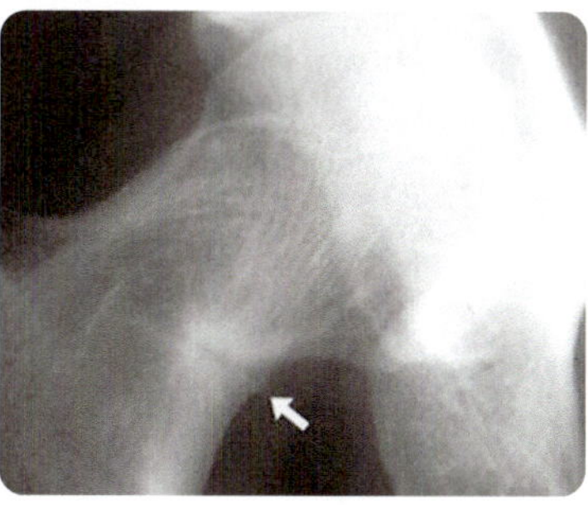

Fig. 3.1.5: Looser zone (arrow) seen in the femoral neck of a patient with osteomalacia.

DDx

- Primary hyperparathyroidism
- Osteoporosis
- Multiple myeloma
- Paget's disease

Management

General measures:

- Treat the **underlying cause**.
- **Adequate safe exposure to sunlight**.
- **Adequate dietary intake of vitamin D** – foods such as oily fish / cod liver oil, egg yolk and milk are rich in vitamin D. Some foods are supplemented with vitamin D, such as breakfast cereals.
- **Daily vitamin D and calcium tablets, e.g. Adcal D_3**.

Box 3.1.2: Implications of vitamin D deficiency / insufficiency

Vitamin D deficiency is also associated with adverse health risks including:

- ↑ risk of **type 2 diabetes mellitus**
- ↑ risk of **several cancers**, e.g. prostate cancer
- ↑ risk of **cardiovascular disease**

Supplementation:

In patients with developed vitamin deficiency (25-(OH)D <30 nmol/L), high-dose supplementation is needed to achieve adequate vitamin D replacement (*Table 3.1.2*). Calcium intake should also be assessed. Local guidelines should be followed.

Table 3.1.2: High-dose vitamin D supplementation in children and adults

Children	Adults
<6 months old – **3000 IU oral calciferol daily** for **8–12 weeks** with calcium supplementation, followed by **200–400 IU calciferol** daily maintenance.	**4000 IU calciferol daily** or **50 000 IU calciferol weekly** for **6–10 weeks (300 000 IU over total course)** followed by **800–2000 IU calciferol daily maintenance** (10 000 IU weekly) (NICE, 2018).
>6 months old – **6000 IU oral calciferol** daily for **8–12 weeks** followed by **400–600 IU calciferol daily**.	Patients with severe malabsorption are treated with higher doses, e.g. **intramuscular calciferol 300 000 IU monthly for 3 months** and then yearly maintenance doses (this can be increased up to 4000 IU daily following specialist advice).

Self-assessment

A 2 year old girl has failure to thrive and an unusual gait. She has bowed legs and thick wrists. Her weight and height are below that expected for her age. Her diet consists predominantly of breastfeeding 5 times daily. Laboratory studies reveal the 25-hydroxyvitamin D level is decreased.

1. What condition is this girl suffering from?
2. What is the likely cause of her condition?
3. What further blood tests may you request and what might they show?
4. What abnormalities do you expect to see on X-ray of her wrists and knees?
5. Her parents are extremely worried. How would you reassure them?

Answers to self-assessment questions are to be found on the Resources tab at www.scionpublishing.com/Rheum2.

3.2 Juvenile idiopathic arthritis

Juvenile idiopathic arthritis (JIA) is a heterogeneous disease with several subtypes defined as any chronic (≥**6 weeks**) **arthritis** affecting individuals **under the age of 16 years** with other known conditions excluded. It is characterized by joint inflammation, pain and stiffness that can lead to joint damage and disability if left untreated.

Pathophysiology

- The pathophysiology of JIA is poorly understood.
- Monozygotic twin concordance (25–40%) indicates the importance of genetic factors.
- Different HLA polymorphisms have been associated with different subtypes of JIA.
- **Systemic JIA** is characterized by **chronic inflammation** of the **synovium** with infiltration of innate inflammatory cells. These then release various pro-inflammatory cytokines (e.g. IL-1, IL-6, IL-17) which result in **increased synovial fluid production** and a **thickened synovial lining**.
- For the oligoarthritis, polyarthritis and psoriatic arthritis subtypes of JIA there is dysregulation of the adaptive immune system leading to imbalances of Treg, Th1 (IFN-γ secreting), and Th17 (IL-17 secreting). This leads to the production of pro-inflammatory cytokines and matrix metalloproteinases causing joint damage.
- In RF-positive JIA, IL-23 causes inflammation and new bone formation through IL-17 and TNF, and IL-22 respectively.
- According to the International League of Associations for Rheumatology (ILAR), JIA can be classified into seven subtypes (*Table 3.2.1*).

Table 3.2.1: ILAR classification of JIA

Sub-group	Prevalence %
1) Oligoarticular JIA	50–60
2) Polyarticular JIA – RF negative	11–28
3) Polyarticular JIA – RF positive	2–7
4) Systemic-onset JIA	10–20
5) Juvenile psoriatic arthritis	2–15
6) Enthesitis-related arthritis	1–7
7) Undifferentiated arthritis	1–10

Epidemiology and risk factors

- Overall prevalence of JIA is estimated to be 43.5 per 100 000 children in the UK.
- The incidence of JIA is 5.6 per 100 000 children in the UK.
- JIA is generally more common in females (2:1).

Table 3.2.2: Risk factors for JIA	
Gender	• More common in girls **(2:1)**.
Age	• More common in children **aged 2–3**.
Genetic	• **HLA-B27 (enthesitis-related)** • **HLA-A2, HLA-DRB1:11, and HLA-DRB1:08 (oligoarticular and RF negative polyarticular)** • **HLADRB1:01 and HLADRB1:04** (RF-positive) • **HLADRB1:01 and DQA1:01** (psoriatic) • **HLADRB1:04 and DRB1:11** (systemic JIA) • The greater number of risk-alleles present confers an earlier age of onset.
Family history	• Family history of **psoriasis** (first-degree relative), **ankylosing spondylitis** and **inflammatory bowel disease**.
Geography	• Certain subtypes are more common to certain regions, e.g. oligoarthritis is more common in southern Europe, whereas RF-negative arthritis is more common in North America.
Environmental factors	• Antibiotic exposure and caesarean deliveries are possible risk factors.
Ethnicity	• JIA more commonly affects Caucasian children.

Clinical presentation

Subtype	Presentation
Oligoarthritis	• ***Definition***: arthritis affecting 1–4 joints in the first 6 months • ***Persisting oligoarthritis***: **>4 joints** affected within **6 months** • ***Extending oligoarthritis***: **<4 joints** affected within **6 months** • More common in young girls (under the age of 6) • Classically presents with one or two swollen joints causing stiffness and reduced range of movement • **ANA** is positive in 70% • There is no systemic upset and RF is negative • Most commonly affects the **knee** and **ankle**, joints are swollen and warm but not typically very painful • Uveitis is common in this subgroup • Prognosis is good for persisting but poor for extending • Disease flares may occur many years later
Polyarticular RF negative	• ***Definition***: **≥5 joints** affected within **6 months** with a **negative rheumatoid factor** • 2 peaks of age: **toddler to preschool age** and **pre-adolescent** • More common in females (ratio 3:1) • Mild fever, weight loss and anaemia are common • May be **asymmetrical** – high risk of uveitis • May be **symmetrical** with both large and small joint swelling • Presents with minimal swelling but increased stiffness • Often destructive in nature • High remission rate (25%)

Subtype	Presentation
Polyarticular RF positive	• ***Definition***: **≥5 joints** affected in the **first 6 months** with a **positive RF** seen on two separate occasions • More common in older girls (>8 years) • Mild fever, weight loss and anaemia are common • Anti-CCP (+ve) is a predictor of significant joint damage • Associated with **HLA-DR4** • **Symmetrical involvement** of **small joints**, particularly the **hands** and **wrists** with swelling and stiffness • **Erosions**, **joint destruction, rheumatoid nodules** and **systemic features**, e.g. fever and lymphadenopathy • Low remission rate (6%)

Systemic arthritis (Still's disease)	• ***Definition***: arthritis with **intermittent** but **daily fever ≥2 weeks**. There must be one or more of the following:
	  • **Maculopapular rash** (salmon colour which quickly fades)
	  • **Lymphadenopathy**
	  • **Hepatomegaly** and/or **splenomegaly**
	  • **Serositis** (pericarditis, pleuritis, peritonitis)
	• Males and females (1:1), usually before **5 years of age**
	• Arthritis only seen at disease onset in 1/3 of children but commonly develops within a few months, usually symmetrical in nature and affecting several joints
	• Recurrence is common
	• **Macrophage activation syndrome (MAS)** is a serious complication of systemic JIA (80% MAS cases are associated with SJIA). It is a massive inflammatory response leading to fever, hepatosplenomegaly, coagulopathy, encephalopathy, pancytopenia, raised liver enzymes and very high ferritin. Its known triggers include viral infections, arthritis flares and medication changes

Juvenile psoriatic arthritis	• ***Definition***: **arthritis and psoriasis or arthritis** plus at least two of:
	  • **Dactylitis**
	  • **Nail pitting** or **onycholysis**
	  • **Psoriasis** in a first-degree relative
	• Female: male ratio (2:1)
	• Mean age of onset 6 years
	• **Asymmetrical arthritis** affecting **small and large joints**
	• Psoriasis usually occurs before arthritis (>50%)
	• Prognosis moderate

Subtype	Presentation

Enthesitis-related JIA	• ***Definition***: **arthritis** or **enthesitis** plus two of:
	  • **Sacroiliac** or **lumbosacral pain**
	  • **HLA-B27-positive** (65–80% of patients)
	  • **Family history of HLA-B27-related disease**
	  • **Acute anterior uveitis or in a first-degree relative**
	  • **History of SpA in a first-degree relative**
	  • Onset in a **male >6 years of age**
	• Male: female ratio (9:1)
	• Usually presents in those over 10 years
	• Asymmetric arthritis in lower extremities (knee, ankle and hip); Achilles tendon is the most affected site
	• Typically responds well to NSAIDs
	• Prognosis is moderate, with increased likelihood of hip replacement in future

Undifferentiated arthritis	• **Does not fulfil criteria in any subtype or fulfils two or more subtypes**

Diagnosis and investigations

Hx

- Symptoms present in all forms of JIA:
  - **Joint symptoms** (pain, dysfunction, stiffness), particularly after sleep or prolonged sitting
  - **Persistent joint swelling**, particularly the knee, ankle, wrist and small joints of the hand
  - **Difficulty chewing**, **asymmetric mouth opening** and **micrognathia** (undersized jaw)
  - **Muscle atrophy**
  - **Flexion contracture deformity**
  - **Synovial hypertrophy**
- See above for specific symptoms of each subtype
- Ask about family history

Ex

- Joints may be warm and swollen, but are not erythematous
- Do not miss out the TMJ and spine on examination!
- Look for extra-articular features

Ix

There are no specific tests since JIA is a clinical diagnosis!

- **Blood tests:**
  - **Inflammatory markers** such as CRP and ESR are often raised
  - **Positive ANA** → ↑ risk of uveitis
  - **RF positive** in polyarticular RF-positive JIA; anti-CCP – (+ve) may indicate poorer prognosis
  - **HLA-B27** positive in enthesitis-related JIA
- **Imaging:**
  - **X-rays** → usually normal in early JIA but useful to exclude trauma or osteomyelitis; may show periarticular osteoporosis, joint space narrowing, bone erosion, joint subluxation and ankyloses in advanced condition
  - **Ultrasound** → may show joint effusion, synovial hypertrophy, enthesitis and erosions (if present)
  - **MRI** → particularly useful for assessing disease activity in patients with long-standing disease and can also be used to assess response to treatment; most sensitive modality for bone erosions and bone marrow oedema.

DDx

- Septic arthritis
- Osteomyelitis
- Reactive and post-infective arthritis
- Trauma
- Mechanical pain
- Acute rheumatic fever
- Macrophage activation syndrome (MAS)*

Clinical facts: General complications of JIA

- **Osteoporosis**
- **Growth restriction** (related to inflammation)
- **Psychosocial**, **behavioural** and **educational difficulties**
- **Side-effects** of medication

Management

Non-pharmacological management

- **Physiotherapy**, **hydrotherapy** and **occupational therapy** to maintain function and prevent deformities.
- Encouragement of physical activity.
- Liaison with school is important.

---

*According to ACR/EULAR/PRINTO 2016 criteria, a febrile patient with known/suspected SJIA can be classified as having MAS if they have ferritin >684 ng/ml, and **at least two** of the following:

- Platelet count $\leq 181 \times 10^9$/L
- Triglycerides >156 mg/dl
- Fibrinogen $\leq$360 mg/dl
- Aspartate aminotransferase >48 units/L.

Pharmacological management

- **NSAIDs** for symptomatic relief but avoid aspirin (due to risk of Reye's syndrome).
- **Steroids**: intra-articular steroids (triamcinolone hexacetonide preferred) for affected joints and topical steroids for eye involvement; systemic glucocorticoids can be used for MAS.
- **Methotrexate** (preferred cDMARD): first-line treatment if multiple joints are affected.
- **bDMARDs** – can include TNF inhibitors, e.g. etanercept/adalimumab, IL-1/6 inhibitors, e.g. tocilizumab and the T-cell inhibitor abatacept. Generally preferred as an earlier management for SJIA and a later management for oligoarthritis.

Surgery

Soft tissue release, osteotomies and **joint replacement** may be helpful.

Self-assessment

A 3 year old girl attends the rheumatology clinic with her parents. Her parents report a presentation of stiffness and limp of several weeks' duration. The onset was insidious and her parents do not recall any specific injury or prior infections. Her parents also mention that one of her knees is swollen and cannot be straightened, but is not particularly painful. No systemic features are reported. Blood tests reveal that she is RF negative and ANA positive.

1. Give 4 differential diagnoses for a child with a limp.
2. What type of JIA is this child most likely to have?
3. Outline a management plan for her.

Answers to self-assessment questions are to be found on the Resources tab at www.scionpublishing.com/Rheum2.

Chapter 4

Investigations

4.1	Blood tests	110
4.2	Immunological tests	116
4.3	Synovial fluid analysis	120
4.4	Imaging	123

4.1 Blood tests

In rheumatology, investigations can aid diagnosis, predict prognosis, assess disease activity and measure response to treatment. Investigations should only be requested when there are clear indications and results are likely to play a role in shaping the patient's management. Routine blood tests are almost always carried out on patients with suspected rheumatic disease and they consist of **full blood count (FBC)**, **inflammatory markers** and **biochemical tests**.

Full blood count

- FBC is the most common blood test used in clinical settings. It is therefore important to be familiar with its practical aspects as well as being able to interpret it.
- It's important to note the normal range of any test is where **95% of the normal healthy population will lie**. This means that there is 5% of the healthy population which will lie outside the 'normal range'.
- Normal ranges may vary depending on **age**, **sex**, **ethnicity** and coexisting medical conditions such as **splenectomy** and **pregnancy**.
- Each report from the laboratory will give the appropriate normal range for age and sex of the patient.
- Ethnicity can affect WBC and platelet count. For Afro-Caribbean or African individuals, the WBC and neutrophil count normal ranges are much lower.

> **OSCE tips:** Venepuncture
>
> - Avoid taking blood samples from the same site as an infusion, in order to avoid haemodilution.
> - Avoid veins that are thrombosed or close to infection sites.
> - Do NOT use the affected arm in mastectomy or stroke.
> - When performing the procedure, do NOT withdraw the plunger on the sample bottles prior to attachment to the needle as this will create a vacuum which may lead to the collapse of the vein.
> - If a blood culture is required, take cultures first before other blood tests. Blood cultures require a top-notch sterile technique to avoid false positive results.

- FBC blood is usually taken by venepuncture, collected in an EDTA bottle (lavender cap), mixed well and analysed by the laboratory within 4 hours from collection.
- FBC test can be divided into three categories (**red cell parameters**, **white cells** and **platelets**).

Red cell parameters

- **Haemoglobin (Hb) concentration** defines whether the patient is anaemic or not. The normal range of Hb for **men is 130–180 g/L** and **120–160 g/L for women**. Inflammatory rheumatic diseases may result in anaemia (low Hb level). Severe anaemia is considered <80 g/L.
- Hb may be lowered temporarily in patients with RA who are pregnant (up to 100 g/L).
- **Mean cell volume (MCV)** is a mean measure of red cell size and defines the type of anaemia: **macrocytic** (high MCV), **normocytic**, or **microcytic** (low MCV). See *Table 4.1.1*.
- **Mean cell haemoglobin (MCH)** is a measure of the amount of haemoglobin per cell and indicates iron-deficiency anaemia, if low. Patients with rheumatic disease often have a normocytic normochromic anaemia (so-called 'anaemia of chronic disease').

Table 4.1.1: Types of anaemia encountered in rheumatology

Type of anaemia	Blood results	Differential diagnosis
Microcytic anaemia	↓ Hb ↓ MCV ↓ MCH ↓ (Possible) Fe ↓ (Possible) low ferritin ↑ RDW	Chronic blood loss, e.g. bleeding Peptic ulcer due to NSAIDs or steroids Iron deficiency Thalassaemia / sickle cell trait / anaemia
Macrocytic anaemia	↓ Hb ↑ MCV ↓ Possibly folate ↓ Possibly vitamin B_{12}	Azathioprine Methotrexate Excess alcohol consumption Pernicious anaemia Folate/B_{12} deficiency Hypothyroidism
Normocytic anaemia	↓ Hb → MCV ↓ Fe or ↑ Fe or ← Fe ↓ Erythropoietin	Anaemia of chronic disease, e.g. RA and SLE Acute blood loss Mixed picture of micro- and macrocytic anaemia

- **Haematocrit (Hct)**, also known as **packed cell volume (PCV)**, is the volume in percentage (%) of red blood cells in blood (*Fig. 4.1.1*). It is decreased in anaemia, increased by erythrocytosis and influenced by plasma volume. Normal values are 40–54% in men and 36–48% in women.
- **Red cell distribution width (RDW)** measures the range of cell sizes in a sample of blood. Usually red blood cells are a standard size. However, certain disorders (not rheumatological), can cause significant variation in cell size. A higher percentage value indicates a greater distribution of red cell size.

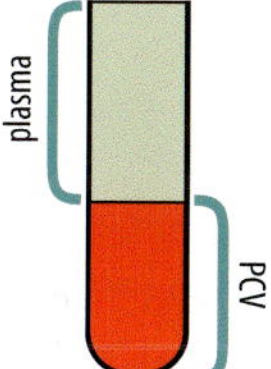

Fig. 4.1.1: Haematocrit or packed cell volume (PCV) illustration.

Other parameters such as **reticulocytes**, **erythropoietin**, **serum iron (Fe)**, **ferritin** (intracellular protein that stores iron), **folate** and **vitamin B_{12} level** are not part of routine FBC and should be requested if required.

White cells

Table 4.1.2: White cell count interpretation

	Raised	Decreased
Neutrophils	**Septic arthritis** caused by bacterial infections, **gout and CPPD**, and **systemic corticosteroids** **Chronic inflammatory disease: SLE, RA** **Smoking**	**SLE, Felty's syndrome** in RA (rare); **Drug-induced**, e.g. DMARDs and **folate deficiency**
Lymphocytes	Viral infection Hyposplenism	Common in **SLE, may also be seen in RA and Sjögren's**
Eosinophils	**Primary vasculitis**, especially Churg–Strauss syndrome associated with asthma / allergy; **polyarteritis nodosa**	Glucocorticoids
Other immune cell counts such as monocyte and basophil count are used less in rheumatology		

Platelets

- **Thrombocytosis**: indicates active inflammation, e.g. RA.
- **Thrombocytopenia**: can be associated with SLE and RA (Felty's syndrome).

Inflammatory markers

Inflammatory markers are usually raised during the **acute phase response**. Two main inflammatory markers are used in rheumatology:

Erythrocyte sedimentation rate (ESR)

- A **non-specific test**.
- The investigation works by assessing how fast red blood cells fall (due to the gravity and high density of RBCs compared to plasma) through a vertical column of anti-coagulated blood in 1 hour (*Fig. 4.1.2*). There is a tendency for RBCs to form clumps ('rouleaux formation'). Clumped RBCs fall faster as they are heavier.
- The rate is measured in **mm/hr** and depends on three factors:
  - **Erythrocytes**: these cells are negatively charged and they tend to repel each other, causing a delay in their settlement. Therefore size, charge and the number of erythrocytes in the blood affect ESR.
  - **Plasma**: acute phase proteins and serum immunoglobulins are large macromolecules that tend to get between erythrocytes, reducing the repulsion forces and increasing the tendency to form rouleaux stacks which increase ESR. During inflammation, serum fibrinogen and immunoglobulin increase, causing ESR to rise.
  - **Technical factors**: laboratory technique and delay in analysis.

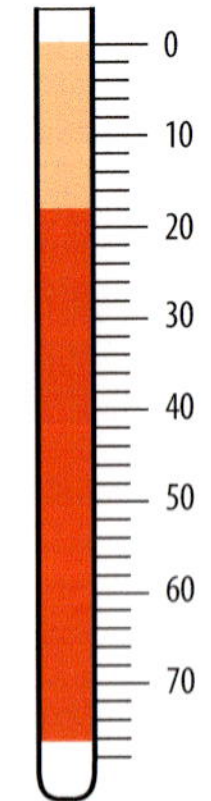

Fig. 4.1.2: RBCs settle after 1 hour, leaving plasma at the top of the tube. The ESR reading is 18 mm/hour.

- In rheumatology, any inflammatory condition, such as **RA**, **GCA** and **PMR**, can cause raised ESR (see *Table 4.1.3* for normal values).
- It is important to note that factors other than inflammation can also result in increased ESR, e.g. **anaemia**, **MI** and **multiple myeloma**. The test should be performed within 2 hours of collection for accurate results.

Table 4.1.3: Normal ESR range (mm/hr) (should be established by lab performing test)

Age	Male	Female
Child	≤10	≤10
17–50	≤15	≤20
50+	≤20	≤30

Note: An easy method to quickly determine if ESR is within the upper limit of normal is by using this formula: normal ESR = male: ≤age/2; female: ≤(age+10)/2. This provides a rough estimate for ESR and does not replace the formal testing required.

C-reactive protein (CRP)

- Any tissue injury or activation of the immune system (e.g. due to an **autoimmune condition or infection**) causes a release of **interleukin-6 (IL-6)**.
- Increases in circulating IL-6 levels stimulate the production and release of CRP and fibrinogen from the liver within **10 hours** of the onset of **inflammation** (*Fig. 4.1.3*). Levels also tend to fall relatively quickly after the removal of the inflammatory stimulus.
- The function of CRP is very similar to immunoglobulins:
  - CRP activates the **complement system** through the classical pathway.
  - CRP activates phagocytic cells via Fc receptor.
  - CRP acts as an **opsonin** for various pathogens.
- CRP is more useful in **monitoring disease activity** and **measuring response to treatment** than for diagnosis.
- CRP can be falsely decreased by NSAIDs and statins. Certain comorbidities can raise CRP, e.g. obesity, insomnia, cancer and depression. Persistently raised CRP may reflect increased cardiovascular risk.

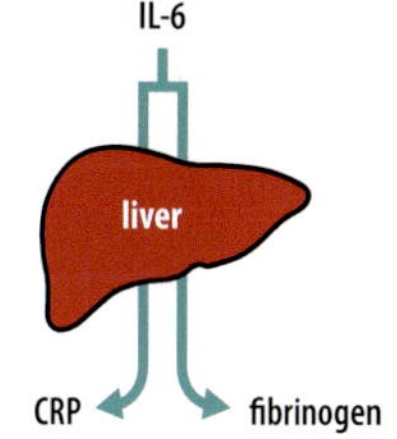

Fig. 4.1.3: CRP release pathway.

Complement test

- Complement components are acute phase proteins.
- Commonly C3/4 measured. This is done at the same time to provide an indication of how each pathway is functioning. A low complement level may indicate active disease.
- May be used to monitor autoimmune diseases, particularly SLE, RA and AxSpA.

Biochemical tests

Biochemical tests are performed in rheumatology for three main reasons:

- To **assess the degree of systemic involvement**, e.g. the use of renal function tests in vasculitis.
- To **monitor adverse drug effects**, e.g. LFTs in patients prescribed methotrexate and DMARDs.
- To **aid diagnosis of certain conditions**, e.g. uric acid measurement in patients with suspected gout.

Liver function tests (LFT)

LFTs are a group of tests that detect any liver damage or disease and they include:

- **Alanine transaminase (ALT), aspartate transaminase (AST)**: increased serum levels may indicate **acute liver damage** (e.g. SLE-associated hepatitis, or hepatitis B leading to secondary vasculitis). They can also indicate **drug-induced hepatitis**, mainly dose related (e.g. **cDMARDs (methotrexate), bDMARDs (tocilizumab), and JAKi (baricitinib)**). It is therefore very important to routinely monitor liver tests in all patients receiving DMARDs.
- **Alkaline phosphatase (ALP):** mainly produced by bile duct cells or **osteoblast cells**. In rheumatology, ALP is markedly raised in **Paget's disease** or in PBC (can be associated with SSC/Sjögren's) and may also be raised in **rickets / osteomalacia** or **bone cancer**.
- **Albumin and total protein**: **SLE** usually causes a decrease in serum albumin level due to glomerulonephritis.
- Other LFT tests such as bilirubin, gamma-glutamyltransferase (GGT), lactate dehydrogenase (LDH) and prothrombin time (PT) are used to a lesser extent in rheumatology.

Renal function tests (RFT)

- There are two reasons to request RFTs in rheumatology:
  - To assess the **extent to which rheumatic diseases affect the kidney** (e.g. SLE and vasculitis).
  - To assess and **monitor the nephrotoxic side-effects** of many drugs used in rheumatology.
- The **eGFR (estimated glomerular filtration rate)** is generally considered to be the best index of kidney function.
- Measuring **plasma creatinine levels** is an inexpensive, quick and widely used method of assessing renal function. Creatinine measurement is a less sensitive measure of renal function than eGFR.
- **Plasma urea** and **electrolyte levels** are an alternative way to assess kidney function. However, levels are less sensitive and specific than eGFR and creatinine plasma level, and many other conditions can influence the results.
- A helpful test in addition to blood testing is **urine dipstick** which may be useful to identify haematuria and proteinuria, which may indicate renal complications from rheumatic disease (lupus nephritis, vasculitis, scleroderma).

Uric acid

- 90% of patients with gout have elevated plasma uric acid levels prior to an acute attack of gout.
- It must be noted, however, that plasma uric acid levels may be normal or fall during an acute attack of gout and therefore their diagnostic use in acute gout is limited.
- Plasma uric acid levels are very useful in measuring disease activity and response to treatment in those with chronic gout.
- Elevated uric acid can also occur in healthy individuals.
- Therefore, the **definitive diagnosis** of gout is based on the presence of **uric acid crystals in synovial fluid**, though this is invasive and therefore not clinically necessary unless there is diagnostic uncertainty.

Tuberculosis test

- bDMARDs may lead to the reactivation of TB and, therefore, should be tested for in all patients prior to initiation.
- Latent TB is commonly assessed for by tuberculin test or interferon-γ release assays.

Bone biochemistry

- There are 3 tests used to assess 3 main rheumatologic bone diseases (osteoporosis, osteomalacia / rickets, and Paget's disease; *Table 4.1.4*):
    1. **Bone-specific alkaline phosphatase** – if high, suspect Paget's disease or osteomalacia.
    2. **Calcium and phosphate plasma level** – if low, suspect osteomalacia.
    3. **Vitamin D** – reduced in rickets and osteomalacia.

Table 4.1.4: Interpretation of bone biochemistry in rheumatology

Condition	Calcium	Phosphate	Alkaline phosphatase	Parathyroid hormone
Osteoporosis	Normal	Normal	Normal	Normal
Osteomalacia and rickets	↓	↓	↑	↑
Paget's disease of bone	Normal	Normal	↑	Normal

4.2 Immunological tests

- Immunological tests play a crucial part in rheumatology, both in terms of providing diagnostic and prognostic value.
- It's important to understand the concept of specificity and sensitivity of diagnostic tests, particularly when it comes to immunological tests:
  - **Sensitivity**: the proportion of people that have the disease and test positive for it. For example, if 90% of patients with RA have a positive test for rheumatoid factor (RF), the sensitivity of RF for detecting RA is 90%.
  - **Specificity**: the proportion of people that don't have the disease and test negative for it. For example, if 98% of patients without RA test negative for anti-CCP, then the specificity of anti-CCP for RA is 98%.
- *Table 4.2.1* summarizes the main immunological tests used in rheumatology.

Table 4.2.1: Immunological tests used in rheumatology

Antibody	Clinical use	Sensitivity (%)	Specificity (%)
Rheumatoid factor (RF)	Aids diagnosis and prognosis of **RA**	**62–87**	**70–96**
Anti-CCP / ACP antibody	Aids diagnosis and prognosis of **RA**	**53–71**	**96**
c-ANCA (antineutrophil cytoplasmic antibodies (cytoplasmic))	Aids diagnosis and prognosis of **Wegener's granulomatosis**	**75**	**98**
p-ANCA (antineutrophil cytoplasmic antibodies (perinuclear))	Aids diagnosis and prognosis of **microscopic polyangiitis**	**46**	**91**
Antinuclear antibody (ANA)	Aids diagnosis of **SLE**	**96**	**81**
Anti-histone antibody	Aids diagnosis of drug-induced lupus erythematosus (DIL) (hydralazine and procainamide rather than bDMARDs)	**67**	**95**
Anti-double-stranded DNA (dsDNA)	Aids diagnosis of **SLE** and provides measurement of disease activity	**37–75**	**94**
Anti-topoisomerase (anti-Scl-70) (extractable nuclear antigen antibodies (ENA))	Aids diagnosis and prognosis of **systemic scleroderma**	**85**	**19**

Table 4.2.1: Immunological tests used in rheumatology *(continued)*

Antibody	Clinical use	Sensitivity (%)	Specificity (%)
Anti-Jo-1 (ENA)	Aids diagnosis and prognosis of **polymyositis**	**20–40**	**Not available**
Anti-Ro (aka anti-SSA) (ENA)	Aids diagnosis of Sjögren's syndrome	**8–70**	**87**
Anti-La (aka anti-SSB) (ENA)	Aids diagnosis of Sjögren's syndrome	**56**	**96**
Anti-SM (ENA)	Aids diagnosis of SLE	**24**	**98**
Anti-RNP (ENA)	Typically found with anti-SM antibodies and associated with several connective tissue diseases	**95–99**	
Anti-chromatin (ENA)	Aids diagnosis of SLE and DIL	**50–100**	**90–99**
Anti-Th/To	Aids diagnosis of CREST syndrome	**27**	**89**
Anti-mitochondrial antibody (AMA)	Aids diagnosis of primary biliary cirrhosis in association with Sjögren's or systemic sclerosis	**84**	**98**
Cardiolipin antibodies (IgG, IgM)	Aids diagnosis of antiphospholipid syndrome and SLE	**40** (IgG) **92** (IgM)	**82.5** (IgG) **1.2** (IgM)
Anti-centromere antibody (ACA)	Aids diagnosis of limited systemic sclerosis (CREST syndrome)	**31**	**97**

Rheumatoid factor

- Ordered when patient has any three criteria for RA (*Sec. 2.1*).
- The timing of RF (+ve) and the titres in patients may indicate more severe disease.
- Targets FC fragment of IgG.
- Testing for RF is cheap and **in the presence of appropriate clinical features it supports the diagnosis of RA**.
- It **does NOT provide a definitive diagnosis on its own**: 15–20% of individuals who are seropositive for RF are in fact healthy, so it should not be used as a general screening tool.
- Other conditions that are seropositive for RF include: **Sjögren's syndrome**, **SLE**, **subacute bacterial endocarditis**, **acute viral infection** and **tuberculosis**.

Anti-cyclic citrullinated peptide (anti-CCP, ACPA) antibodies

- A highly **specific** test (93–98%) for diagnosing RA.
- Excellent in **detecting early disease**; can be positive several years before the onset of RA.
- Targeted against citrulline on proteins.
- RA criteria include the use of **both** RF and anti-CCP.
- Anti-CCP (+ve) can predict erosive joint damage in RA.
- Testing for anti-CCP is expensive; it **costs more** than twice as much as RF.
- The test has the advantage of diagnosing an atypical presentation of RA.
- The test can be positive in other conditions such as Lyme disease, psoriatic arthritis and SLE.

Antineutrophil cytoplasmic antibodies (ANCA)

- Aids the diagnosis of specific subtypes of vasculitis:
  - **Wegener's granulomatosis**: antibodies targeted against proteinase 3 (PR3) → ELISA staining will show **c-ANCA pattern** (*Fig. 4.2.1a*).
  - **Microscopic polyangiitis**: antibodies targeted against myeloperoxidase (MPO) → ELISA staining will show **p-ANCA pattern** (*Fig. 4.2.1b*).
- A rise in ANCA can indicate relapse of the condition.
- Other conditions associated with ANCA are **Churg–Strauss syndrome** and **anti-GBM disease**.

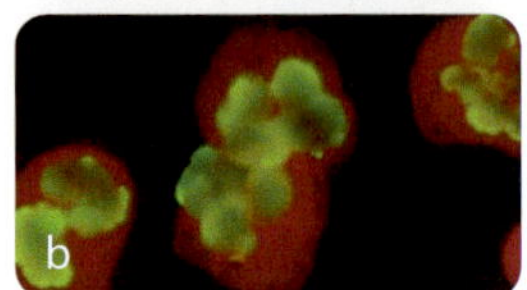

Fig. 4.2.1: (a) Cytoplasmic (c-ANCA); **(b)** perinuclear (p-ANCA).

Antinuclear antibodies (ANA)

- ANA are targeted against cellular components within the nucleus. As such there are many subtypes of ANA antibodies including **anti-dsDNA, anti-Scl-70, anti-Smith, anti-Jo-1** and **anti-Ro** autoantibodies.
- The ANA test is a generic test looking for any positive subtypes. Further tests might be required to confirm the presence of a particular subtype.
- It is the most **sensitive** test (up to 95%) to establish the diagnosis of SLE **in the presence of a typical SLE clinical picture** and is an entry criterion for SLE classification (2019 ACR/EULAR criteria).
- The ANA test has **low specificity** (57%) for SLE; therefore it should only be ordered when the patient fulfils at least **three clinical criteria for SLE** (*Box 2.12.1*).
- Can be positive in healthy individuals (up to 30%) as well as other conditions such as infection (Epstein–Barr virus and viral hepatitis) and neoplastic disease (leukaemia, lymphoma and melanoma).
- ANA can be useful in diagnosing other conditions such as **systemic sclerosis**, with a sensitivity of 85% and a specificity of 54% for picking up the condition.
- Results are reported in titre (e.g. 1:40, 1:60); the higher the titre, the more positive the test is. This is measured using indirect immunofluorescence through a 'fluorescence microscope'.
- Can be split into two categories: antibodies to DNA and histones, and antibodies to additional extractable targeted nuclear antigens (ENA).
- Seropositive results will require further investigation, especially anti-dsDNA test to confirm diagnosis of SLE.

Anti-double-stranded DNA (anti-dsDNA)

- Highly associated with SLE; has a **sensitivity of 57%** and a **specificity of 97%**. Increase in titres tends to occur concomitantly with SLE flares.
- Antibodies targeted against double-stranded DNA (present due to incomplete removal after cell apoptosis) and are mostly detected by immunofluorescence assay.
- Can (very rarely) be positive in other autoimmune conditions such as **RA**, **Sjögren's syndrome**, **chronic active hepatitis**, **uveitis** and **Graves' disease**.

Extractable nuclear antigen antibodies (ENA)

- **Anti-Jo-1**
  - Although they are classified as ANAs, they are usually located in the cytoplasm.
  - Commonly found in patients with **idiopathic inflammatory myopathies**.
  - Found in 20–30% of patients with polymyositis, often in conjunction with **interstitial lung disease** (60–70%).
- **Anti-topoisomerase (anti-Scl-70)**
  - Very practical in diagnosing and predicting the prognosis of **systemic sclerosis**, especially in **diffuse disease**.
  - Antibodies disrupt DNA replication by targeting topoisomerase I.
  - Usually associated with **lung fibrosis** and **renal disease** in systemic sclerosis.
  - **Limited disease (CREST syndrome)** is more closely associated with **anti-centromere antibody (ACA)**, with sensitivity and specificity of 31% and 97%, respectively.
- **Anti-Ro (anti-SSA) and anti-La (anti-SSB)**
  - Associated with increased severity in **primary Sjögren's**.
  - Suspected to target viral DNA of EBV and later cause autoimmune disease.
  - Ro, like Jo-1, is typically found outside the nucleus. However, La is usually found within the nucleus.
  - Can also be positive in other conditions such as **SLE** and **neonatal lupus**.
- **Anti-Smith (Sm)**
  - The Smith antigen is an SLE antigen (RNA binding protein complex) that is present in up to 30% of patients.
  - Measured through radioactive immunoassay.
  - Highly specific for lupus (98%).
- **Anti-Th/To**
  - Used to aid diagnosis of SSc and of particular value in diagnosing related-ILD.
  - Can also be positive in RA, SLE, Sjögren's and ITP.
- **Anti-centromere**
  - Target autoantibodies specific to centromere.
  - Can be detected in patients with SS, SSc and primary biliary cholangitis.

4.3 Synovial fluid analysis

Synovial fluid consists of a transudate of plasma from synovial blood vessels, supplemented with saccharide-rich molecules. The function of synovial fluid is to provide nutrients to the cartilage and to act as a lubricant. The volume and characteristics of synovial fluid change in response to trauma, infection and inflammation.

Arthrocentesis (joint aspiration)

- Fluid is collected by needle aspiration, sometimes in conjunction with ultrasound, CT or fluoroscopy for deeper joints. This can be for analysis or therapeutically if there is an effusion impacting on range of movement and/or causing pain.
- Normal fluid will not clot; however, fluid from a diseased joint may contain fibrinogen, causing it to clot.
- An ethylenediaminetetraacetic acid (EDTA) tube is used to collect fluid for cell count, a heparinized tube for chemical and immunological tests, and a sterile tube for microbiological testing and crystal examination.
- Indications, contraindications and complications are summarized in *Table 4.3.1*.

Table 4.3.1: Indications, contraindications and complications of arthrocentesis

Indications	• To establish the underlying cause of an acute monoarthritis or polyarthritis which include:
	  • septic arthritis – which must not be missed as it can lead to irreversible joint destruction
	  • other conditions such as crystal arthropathies, rheumatic disorders and haemarthrosis
	• Arthrocentesis is also used to drain large effusions (including septic causes, or from chronic arthritis) or haemarthrosis to relieve pain

Contraindications	• Cellulitis (seeding infection within joint) • Prosthetic joint (should be referred to an orthopaedic surgeon) • Patients with coagulopathy or who are on anticoagulants – consider reversing anticoagulation before procedure to reduce risk of haemarthrosis
Complications	• These include iatrogenic infection, localized trauma, pain, and reaccumulation of the effusion.

Characteristics of normal synovial fluid

- An ultra-filtrate of plasma which is clear, or pale yellow and transparent (*Fig. 4.3.1*).
- Absence of clotting factors.
- Viscous fluid.
- Absence of inflammatory cells.
- Lack of particulates (small particles).

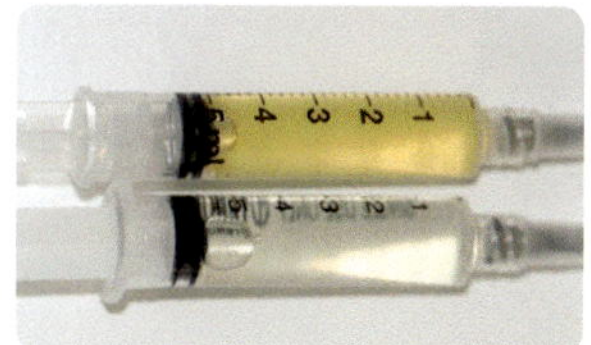

Fig. 4.3.1: (Top) yellow opaque synovial fluid; (Bottom) normal synovial fluid (see *Table 4.3.1* for causes).

The synovial fluid examination (*Table 4.3.2*)

- Evaluation of the **appearance of fluid: colour** (cells, fibrin and depolymerized macromolecules increase intensity), clarity (not standardized), volume and **viscosity** (drop test).
- **Cell count** for inflammatory and haemorrhagic pathology. The gold-standard measurement is cells per cubic millimetre, calculated by doing a manual cell count. After a total WBC count has been completed, a differential cell count can be done to confirm or rule out diagnoses.
- **Microscopic examination** for particulates:
  - Gout → **monosodium urate crystals** showing **negative birefringence** under polarized light microscopy (*Fig. 4.3.2a*).
  - CPPD → **CPP crystals** showing **positive birefringence under polarized light microscopy** (*Fig. 4.3.2b*).
- **Microbiology tests (Gram stain** and **culture)** for septic arthritis.
- **Chemical laboratory**:
  - **Glucose** → usually decreased in septic arthritis.
  - **Protein** and **LDH** → usually increased in RA, septic arthritis and gout.

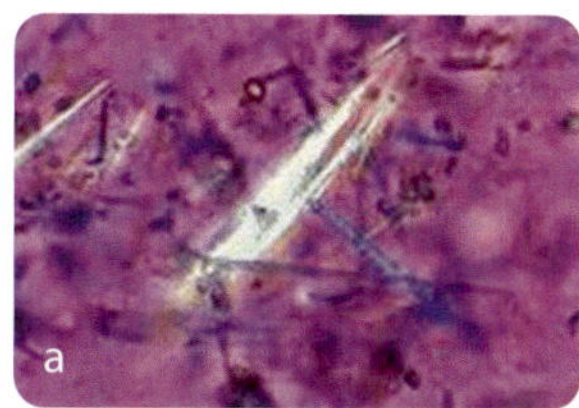

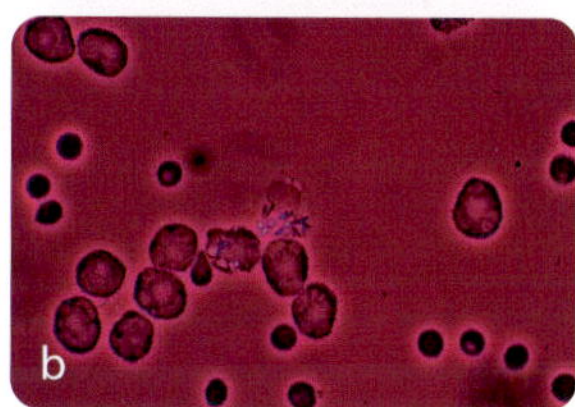

Fig. 4.3.2: (**a**) Needle-shaped monosodium urate crystals; (**b**) rhomboidal CPP crystals.

Table 4.3.2: Synovial fluid interpretation

	Normal	Non-inflammatory	Inflammatory	Microbial infection	Crystal pathology	Haemorrhagic
Disease		**OA**	**RA, SLE**	**Septic arthritis**	**Gout and CPPD**	**Traumatic injury**
Clarity	Transparent	Transparent	Cloudy	Opaque	Cloudy	Bloody
Colour	Clear	Yellow	Yellow	Yellow	Yellow	Red
Viscosity	High	High	Low	Variable	Variable	Variable
WBC count/ mm^3	<200	200–2000	2000–50 000	>20 000 Typically over 50 000; however, in gonococcal infection or if on antibiotics this may be lowered	Gout: 100–160 000 CPPD: 3000–100 000	200–2000
Neutrophils (%)	<25	<25	RA 50–75 SLE <25	>75 (if bacterial)	~90	<50
Other features			RA may have decreased levels of glucose. RA and SLE have elevated levels of RF.	Septic arthritis can have decreased levels of glucose. A negative Gram stain should not exclude septic arthritis.	Presence of CPP or uric acid crystals.	

4.4 Imaging

- There are different imaging modalities that can aid clinicians in diagnosing, managing and monitoring rheumatological conditions.
- These imaging modalities include **X-ray**, **ultrasound scan (USS)**, **computed tomography (CT)**, **magnetic resonance imaging (MRI)**, **dual-energy X-ray absorptiometry (DEXA)**, and sometimes **scintigraphy**.
- It is important to have a framework to work through before requesting imaging.

Before making any **referral request** ask yourself five questions:

1. Has it been done already?
2. Do I have a question the investigation will answer?
   - Are there early signs of inflammation?
   - Where is the location of inflammation?
   - Will this reduce the differential diagnosis?
   - Is this likely to affect the management plan?
3. Do I need it now?
   - Some imaging processes may take longer than others.
4. Is this the best investigation?
   - Pros and cons; are there alternatives that may be better suited?
5. Are there any contraindications? (see *OSCE tips*, below)

Once you or your consultant decide to make a referral, make sure you complete a request form to effectively communicate with the imaging department. Ensure the following details are included:

- **Patient's demographic details: name, d.o.b., address, pregnancy status, interpreting needs** and **hospital ID**.
- **Patient's clinical status** and whether it's **urgent** or not.
- **Patient's mobility**: positioning of some imaging techniques require the patient to be mobile.
- **Patient location and travel details**: which ward to escort from and return to, any need to maintain the patient under specific therapy (e.g. oxygen) during the imaging procedure.
- **Contact details**: this includes names (yours and your consultant's), department and telephone / bleep number.
- **Clinical information**: this should show the rationale behind the request, which should include the indications and any contraindications.

OSCE tips: Imaging contraindications

- **Pregnancy and radiation**: any female of childbearing age should be asked whether there is any chance that she could be pregnant and to sign a declaration for this. History of last menstrual period must be taken. This is particularly relevant for imaging that involves radiation such as X-rays or CT scans.
- **Intravenous (IV) contrast**: these are nephrotoxic chemicals and therefore renal function tests should be performed before proceeding with imaging that uses IV contrast.
- **Patients can be allergic to IV contrasts**: therefore ask about allergies and previous IV contrast procedure complications (if any).
- **Magnetic resonance imaging**: metallic foreign bodies (FBs) in the orbits, aneurysm clips, pacemakers and cochlear implants.

X-ray

X-rays consist of ionizing radiation that passes through the body and is variably attenuated depending on the structure it passes through:

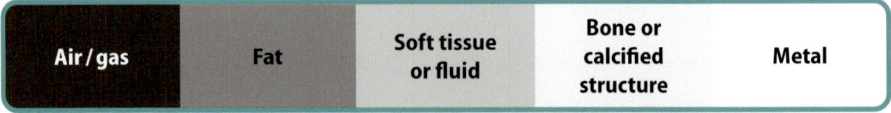

Air / gas	Fat	Soft tissue or fluid	Bone or calcified structure	Metal

- **Inexpensive** and **readily available**.
- Can show joint damage such as **bone erosion** or **cartilage damage** (joint space narrowing) which can aid the diagnosis of arthritis (see *OSCE tips*, below).
- These changes tend to occur in the **later stages of disease**; early changes are often not picked up on plain radiography.
- Can be **useful in management**: chest X-ray is recommended before starting methotrexate treatment and requested yearly (depending on symptoms) to check for methotrexate-induced pneumonitis.

OSCE tips: Presenting X-ray checklist!

1. Patient name, gender, d.o.b. and hospital ID
2. Date on which X-ray was taken
3. Comment on the technical aspects:
    - **Orientation** (confirm by the marker (left or right))
    - **X-ray projection**: PA, AP or lateral
    - **Rotation** (if any)
    - **Penetration** (adequate or non-adequate)
4. Describe the visible anatomy **systematically**
5. At the end, summarize the findings in one sentence
6. Offer differential diagnosis

OSCE tips: RA vs OA X-ray changes

RA	OA
Narrowing of joint space	Narrowing of joint space
Periarticular osteopenia	Osteophytes
Juxta-articular bony erosions	Subchondral cysts
Subluxation and gross deformity	Subchondral sclerosis
Periarticular soft tissue swelling	Chondrocalcinosis

Ultrasound scan (USS)

- **A dynamic real-time imaging modality** that utilizes ultrasound (1–15 MHz) as an emission source.
- The ultrasound (US) travels through the body at different velocities (depending on the density) and is reflected.
- The image is constructed based on the amount and timing of the reflected US.
- Widely used in rheumatology for:
    - **detecting synovitis**
    - **detecting joint effusion**: it is possible to detect even small effusions

  - **assessing cartilage degeneration and bone erosion**
  - **assessing blood vessels**: may show vessel oedema in giant cell arteritis
  - **guiding joint injection** or **aspiration**.
- **Advantages of US include**: inexpensive, non-invasive, non-radioactive, portable and quick.
- **Disadvantages of US**: operator dependent and interpretation of static image can be difficult (generally more useful for more superficial joints).

Computed tomography (CT)

- By using a computer, several X-ray images of the body are taken and converted into a 3D picture.
- More sensitive at picking up early inflammatory/subtle changes compared to X-ray.
- Disadvantages: low sensitivity for previewing soft tissue changes and high exposure to ionizing radiation.
- CT scan images can be enhanced using IV contrast agents which are iodine based.
- IV contrast can cause nausea and vomiting, urticaria, renal failure and anaphylaxis.
- **CT is rarely used in rheumatology unless X-ray is unclear and MRI is unavailable**.

Magnetic resonance imaging (MRI)

- Utilizes a magnetic field to align hydrogen nuclei, mainly in the body's water molecules.
- Used in rheumatology for **soft tissue abnormalities**, e.g. in **detecting synovitis**, **tenosynovitis**, **tendon rupture** and **intervertebral disc abnormalities**.
- Also shows bone oedema, which is an early sign of inflammation that is not detected by plain radiography.
- Smaller joints are less well imaged compared to larger joints.
- Contraindicated if there is any **metalwork** in the body.
- **Expensive** and access in the NHS is restricted.
- Can be useful in atypical RA, PsA, and AS.
- Unlike the CT scanner, the MRI scanner is fully enclosed, which can be problematic for patients with **claustrophobia** or **obesity**.

Dual-energy X-ray absorptiometry (DEXA)

- Measures **bone mineral density (BMD)** in **grams of hydroxyapatite/cm^3**.
- DEXA scan is used to diagnose patients with suspected osteoporosis. Interpretation of the result is explained in *Sec. 2.17*.
- DEXA may also be used after the prescription of glucocorticoids to monitor bone health, or in other autoimmune conditions which are associated with osteoporosis.
- Scanning is most often preferred at the **spine** or **hip**.
- Works by directing two low-energy X-ray beams through the bone being tested. The X-ray is then detected on the other side. The denser the bone, the lower the amount of X-ray reaching the detector.

Scintigraphy and FDG (fluorodeoxyglucose) PET scan

- Bone scintigraphy (bone scan) typically occurs in three phases and is often used to show the effectiveness of treatment for synovitis by intra-articular injection of radioactive isotopes (radiosynoviorthesis).
- It may also be helpful in detecting the activity of inflammatory arthritis, as it is highly sensitive (though not specific) in identifying inflammation, with the added benefits of low radiation exposure and cost. Additionally, it is valuable for confirming degenerative arthritis and excluding inflammatory arthritis.
- FDG PET uses F-fluorodeoxyglucose as a tracer. It is typically used for vasculitis where it has some benefits in differentiating large vessel vasculitides from isolated vasculitis.
- FDG PET can also be used to classify GCA (non-cranial) and PMR (EULAR).

Chapter 5

Pharmacology

5.1	Analgesia	128
5.2	Corticosteroids	133
5.3	Osteoporosis drugs	135
5.4	DMARDs and biological agents	139

5.1 Analgesia

- As with many other specialties, pain control plays a central role in rheumatology. It has emotional, cognitive and physical components. It is a unique experience and is multifaceted. Many rheumatological conditions are chronic and affect activities of daily living.
- The analgesic pain ladder is useful for determining which analgesic to use (*Fig. 5.1.1*). However, to address the other components of pain a newer 'trolley' approach is taken. This includes non-invasive therapy as well as drug categories or surgical techniques to be selected at the discretion of the clinician, as opposed to a formulaic stepwise approach.
- Analgesia should be a dynamic treatment such that pain is addressed more holistically. This more personalized approach also allows clinicians to decide the best approach based on factors such as individual response to medication.

Adjuvants

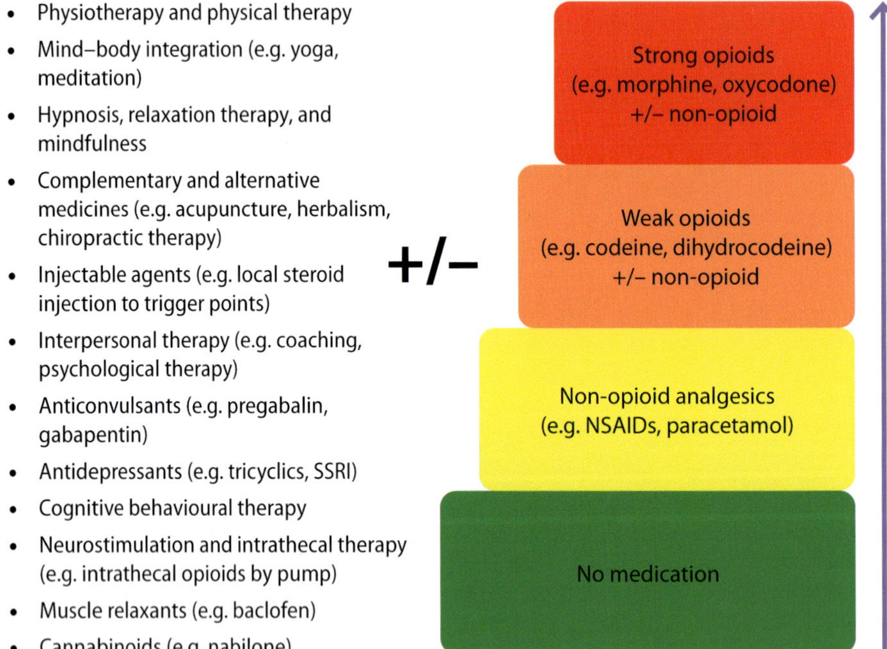

Fig. 5.1.1: Pain platform. The adjuvants are up to the discretion of the clinician to be added or removed on a case-by-case basis.

Paracetamol

- Paracetamol is usually the first-line treatment for mild pain relief and its lack of side-effects and contraindications makes it a very safe agent.

Table 5.1.1: Paracetamol (acetaminophen)

Indications	**Mild / moderate pain** and **fever**
Mechanisms of action	The mechanism of action of paracetamol involves weak suppression of COX enzymes, resulting in reduced production of prostaglandins from arachidonic acid. This therefore controls inflammation, pain and fever. It also is metabolized to form *N*-arachidonoylphenolamine, an endocannabinoid reuptake inhibitor contributing to the activation of the bulbospinal serotonergic pathway.
Side-effects	**Rare:** severe cutaneous adverse skin reactions, blood disorders (including thrombocytopenia, leucopenia, and neutropenia), hypotension, bronchospasm, flushing, tachycardia (on infusion) and liver/renal damage (overdose)
Contraindications	None, but caution in hepatic and renal impairment
Dosage	Max dose may decrease if there is hepatotoxicity By mouth, **0.5–1 g every 4–6 hours**, max. 4 g/24 hours By IV (<51 kg), **15 mg/kg every 4–6 hours administered over 15 minutes**, max. 60 mg/kg/24 hours By IV (>51 kg), **15 mg/kg every 4–6 hours administered over 15 minutes**, max. 4 g/24 hours
Route	**Oral**, **rectal** and **IV**

NSAIDs

- Non-steroidal anti-inflammatory drugs (NSAIDs) contain both **analgesic** and **anti-inflammatory** properties and work by inhibiting the production of **prostaglandins** via inhibition of **COX enzyme**. Anti-inflammatory effects do not vary greatly; however, there is considerable variation in how some patients respond to and tolerate different NSAIDs.
- NSAIDs vary in their selectivity for inhibiting different types of COX (**COX-1 and COX-2**); selective inhibition of COX-2 is associated with less GI intolerance but they have similar efficacy and cardiovascular risk profile (*Fig. 5.1.2*).
- Examples of **non-selective COX inhibitors** include **ibuprofen, naproxen** and **diclofenac**. **Selective COX-2 inhibitors** include **celecoxib, etoricoxib** and **meloxicam**.
- **Topical NSAIDs** (e.g. ibuprofen gel, diclofenac gel) can be applied directly to the site of pain and inflammation, e.g. in OA. Although they are not as strong as oral NSAIDs, topical NSAIDs do not possess the same systemic side-effects or contraindications.

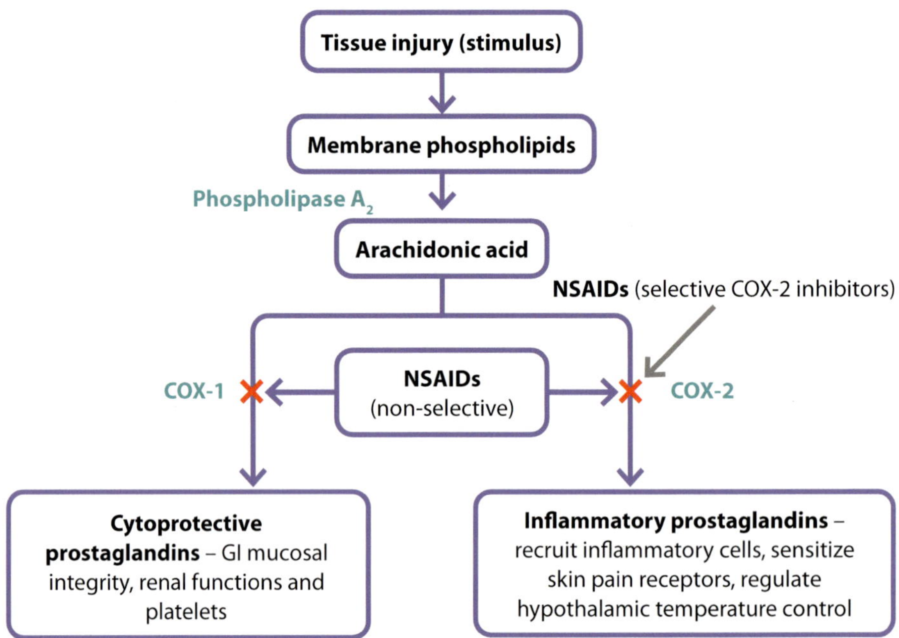

Fig. 5.1.2: The mechanism of action of NSAIDs involves suppression of COX enzymes, resulting in reduced production of prostaglandins from arachidonic acid. This therefore controls inflammation, pain and fever.

Table 5.1.2: NSAIDs

Examples	• Non-selective – **ibuprofen**, **diclofenac**, **naproxen** and **indomethacin** • Selective – **celecoxib**, **meloxicam** and **etoricoxib**.
Indications	To reduce mild / moderate pain and inflammation: **inflammatory arthritis (RA**, **AS**, **PsA)** and **OA**.
Mechanisms of action	See *Fig. 5.1.2.*
Side-effects	Most commonly **GI disturbances** including discomfort, nausea, diarrhoea, and occasionally GI bleeding and ulceration occur; ↑ risk of CVD, hypersensitivity reactions, headache, dizziness, nervousness, depression, drowsiness, insomnia, vertigo, hearing disturbances, worsening of asthma, renal failure, and restriction of fetal growth.
Contraindications	Acute renal failure (ARF), chronic renal failure (CRF), ischaemic heart disease (IHD), congestive cardiac failure (CCF), asthma, pregnancy, breastfeeding, elderly, active bleeding, active or recurrent GI ulcers, history of GI bleeding and coagulopathies. Caution needed for NSAID use and excessive alcohol consumption.

Table 5.1.2: NSAIDs *(continued)*	
Dose	• **Ibuprofen**: initially 300–400 mg 3–4 times daily; max. 2.4 g daily • **Naproxen**: 0.5–1 g daily in 1–2 divided doses • **Diclofenac**: 75–150 mg daily in 2–3 divided doses
Route	• **Ibuprofen**: oral, topical, IV • **Naproxen**: oral • **Diclofenac**: oral, rectal, intramuscular (IM), IV, topical

DO:	DO NOT:
• Consider renal function before placing a patient on NSAIDs. • Inform the patient to take with food and give gastric protection in the form of a PPI or H_2 antagonist if patient is on long-term non-selective NSAIDs. • Tell the patient it may take several weeks for a good NSAID effect.	• Assume that if one NSAID is ineffective, others will be too. Try another class if one doesn't work. • Prescribe NSAIDs without checking for significant contraindications, such as significant asthma, renal failure or history of GI bleed.

Opioids

- Opioid analgesics are used to relieve **moderate to severe pain**.
- **Compound analgesics**, e.g. **co-codamol** and **co-dydramol**, are a combination of first-step analgesics (paracetamol) and a weak opioid (codeine).
- Repeated administration may cause dependence and tolerance, but this is no deterrent in the control of pain in terminal illness.
- Research shows that there may be synergistic effects of paracetamol or NSAIDs with opiates to allow the use of a lower dose / prevent dose escalation.
- When starting strong opioid treatment, e.g. morphine, opioid-induced nausea often responds well to anti-emetic treatment; this should therefore be considered as prophylaxis against nausea.

Table 5.1.3: Opioids	
Examples	**Codeine phosphate** (mild / moderate pain), **tramadol hydrochloride** (moderate / severe pain), **morphine salts**, **fentanyl**, **diamorphine**, and **hydrochloride** (severe pain).
Indications	**Mild–severe pain**
Mechanism of action	Opioids exert their effects through binding to **opioid receptors** – MOP (**μ**), DOP (**δ**), and KOP (**κ**) within the **central and peripheral nervous system** to activate descending inhibitory neurons. This results in a reduction in nociceptive transmission from the periphery. Opioids can also act directly on peripheral nociceptive afferent neurons by preventing the release of neurotransmitters and hyperpolarizing post-synaptic cells. This decreases transmission further.

Table 5.1.3: Opioids *(continued)*	
Side-effects	The most common side-effects include nausea and vomiting (particularly in initial stages), constipation, dry mouth, and biliary spasm; larger doses produce muscle rigidity, dizziness, drowsiness, hypotension, **respiratory depression** (most severe symptom), arrhythmias, hallucinations, withdrawal syndrome and confusion.
Contraindications	Acute respiratory depression, paralytic ileus, raised intracranial pressure and in head injury, comatose patients, hepatic impairment, renal impairment, pregnancy and breastfeeding. Driving should be avoided.
Dose (oral)	• **Codeine phosphate**: **30–60 mg every 6 hours** when necessary, to a max. of 240 mg daily • **Co-codamol**: 30 mg (codeine)/500 mg (paracetamol) or 8/500 mg: 2 tablets every 4–6 hours with a maximum of 8 tablets per day • **Dihydrocodeine phosphate**: 30 mg every 4–6 hours when necessary; this can be increased to 60–120 mg every 12 hours in chronic severe pain • **Tramadol hydrochloride**: 50–100 mg every 4 hours; maximum of 400 mg/24 hrs • **Morphine salts**: see the *BNF*
Routes	• **Codeine phosphate**: oral, IM • **Dihydrocodeine phosphate**: oral, subcutaneous (SC) or IM • **Tramadol hydrochloride**: oral, SC, IM or IV • **Morphine salts**: oral, rectal, IM, SC or IV

DO:	DO NOT:
• Consider co-prescribing a prophylactic anti-emetic when prescribing strong opioids such as morphine. • Consider co-prescribing laxatives to prevent constipation.	• Fail to warn about common and significant side-effects of opioids, such as nausea, constipation and drowsiness. • Fail to recognize signs of opioid-induced toxicity: pinpoint pupils, bradycardia, poor respiratory effort and stridor. Stop opioid and give naloxone if this happens.

5.2 Corticosteroids

- Corticosteroids include glucocorticoids and mineralocorticoids; however, the term generally refers to glucocorticoids.
- Corticosteroids have both **immunosuppressive** and **anti-inflammatory** properties.
- **Prednisolone** is the most commonly used corticosteroid for treating rheumatic disease.
- Corticosteroids (particularly systemic ones) come with a great number of adverse effects.
- **Systemic corticosteroids** are the treatment of choice for **GCA** and **PMR**. Here the aim is to control the disease by maintaining a high steroid dose for a period. Subsequently, the dose may be tapered with a view to stopping altogether if remission has been achieved and sustained.
- **Local steroid injections** can be given for **soft-tissue inflammation** and **OA**.
- **Steroid-sparing agents** (e.g. **azathioprine** or **methotrexate**) are commonly given with steroids to allow for the dose of steroids to be reduced.

Table 5.2.1: Corticosteroids

Examples	Corticosteroids most used in practice; properties values are relative to hydrocortisone.

Drug	Gluco-corticoid properties	Mineralo-corticoid properties	General indication
Hydrocortisone	1	1	Corticosteroid replacement therapy
Prednisolone	4	0.8	Anti-inflammatory and immunosuppressive
Methyl-prednisolone	5	Negligible	Anti-inflammatory and immunosuppressive

Indications	**PMR**, **GCA**, **vasculitis**, **PM** and **DM**, **SLE**, **RA** and **gout**.
Mechanism of action	1. **Anti-inflammatory:** bind to intracellular glucocorticoid receptors to suppress (transrepression) transcription factors related to pro-inflammatory mediator synthesis and related enzymes like phospholipase A_2. 2. **Immunosuppressive:** inhibit T-lymphocytes and reduce neutrophil migration, suppressing delayed hypersensitivity reactions. Suppress COX-2, nitric oxide synthase, and pro-inflammatory cytokine genes (interleukins and TNF-α). 3. **Anti-proliferative:** block DNA synthesis and epidermal cell division. 4. **Vasoconstrictive:** inhibit histamine and other vasoconstrictive mediators and directly affecting vascular endothelial cells.
Side-effects ('CUSHINGOID FAM')	Cushing's syndrome, Cataracts, Ulcers (peptic), Skin (striae, thinning, bruising), Hypertension, Infections, Necrosis, Growth restriction (children), Osteoporosis, Obesity (central), Immunosuppression, Diabetes, Fluid retention, Acute pancreatitis and Myopathy.

Table 5.2.1: Corticosteroids *(continued)*	
Contraindications	**Absolute:** acute uncontrolled infections. **Caution:** liver failure, renal failure, heart failure, acute pancreatitis, diabetes, Cushing's syndrome, peptic ulcers, osteoporosis, psychoses, systemic sclerosis, hypertension, glaucoma, TB, hypothyroidism, ulcerative colitis, diverticulitis, pregnancy, breastfeeding, elderly and children.
Doses (oral prednisolone)	Depends on route and indication. The *BNF* guide recommends: • **RA**: 7.5 mg/daily. • **PMR**: 10–15 mg/daily. Continued until disease activity is controlled, and then doses are gradually reduced to a 7.5–10 mg/daily maintenance. • **GCA**: 40–60 mg/daily gradually reduced to 7.5–10 mg/daily for maintenance. • **Polyarteritis nodosa and PM**: 60 mg/day (initially), then reduced to a maintenance dose of 10–15 mg/daily. • **SLE**: 60 mg/day (initially), then reduced to a maintenance dose of 10–15 mg/daily.
Route	• Prednisolone: oral. • Hydrocortisone: oral, IM and IV.

DO:	DO NOT:
• Prescribe a **bisphosphonate**, e.g. alendronic acid, if on >7.5 mg oral steroids (long-term) to prevent glucocorticoid-induced osteoporosis. • If medium- to long-term therapy is anticipated, bisphosphonate (bone protection) should be started as early as possible. • Give **gastroprotection**, e.g. PPI, for those on long-term corticosteroids. • Give higher maintenance doses during times of concomitant illness and stress (e.g. surgery). • Use lowest possible dose for shortest amount of time.	• Prescribe oral steroids for chronic pain syndromes, or vague aches and pains. • Prescribe oral steroids if 'all else has failed'. • Stop long-term steroids suddenly; it should be tapered gradually.

5.3 Osteoporosis drugs

- Pharmacological agents for osteoporosis are given either to prevent fractures (**primary prevention**) in individuals who are at high risk of fractures, or to prevent further fractures in those who have already had a fracture (**secondary prevention**).
- Osteoporosis agents can be divided into **anabolic treatment (stimulate bone formation) and anti-resorptive treatment**. Some medications have overlapping characteristics (*Fig. 5.3.1*).
- **Bisphosphonates** are usually first-line agents in osteoporosis patients but other effective agents are also available: **raloxifene**, **teriparatide**, **abaloparatide**, **denosumab** and **romosozumab**.

Table 5.3.1: Bisphosphonates

Examples	**Alendronic acid** (alendronate), **ibandronic acid** (ibandronate), **risedronate sodium**, **zoledronic acid** (zoledronate).
Indications	Osteoporosis (first-line), Paget's disease and bone metastases.
Mechanism of action	**Bisphosphonates inhibit osteoclast action.** They impair the ability of the osteoclasts to form the ruffled border and adhere to the bony surface. They also reduce the activity of osteoclasts by decreasing osteoclast progenitor development and recruitment, and by promoting osteoclast apoptosis, thus inhibiting bone resorption. They have some positive effect on osteoblasts, but this is minor in comparison to their osteoclast inhibition. **Bisphosphonates decrease the risk of vertebral and non-vertebral fractures.**
Side-effects	Oesophageal reactions (ulcers, stricture and erosions, and oesophagitis), abdominal pain and distension, constipation, diarrhoea, dizziness, alopecia, anaemia, vomiting, dyspepsia, regurgitation, renal impairment, atypical femur fractures (rare), Stevens–Johnson syndrome (rare), osteonecrosis of the jaw (rare), and osteonecrosis of the external auditory canal (very rare).
Contraindications	Dysphagia, achalasia, stricture, pregnancy, breastfeeding, hypocalcaemia, GI ulceration, inflammation or bleeding, and renal impairment.

Table 5.3.1: Bisphosphonates *(continued)*	
Dose	• **Alendronic acid**: 10 mg/daily or 70 mg/weekly PO (treatment for post-menopausal osteoporosis, osteoporosis in men, and treatment and prevention for corticosteroid-induced osteoporosis). • **Ibandronic acid**: 150 mg/month PO or 3 mg/3 month IV (treatment for post-menopausal osteoporosis). • **Risedronate sodium**: for Paget's disease of bone, 30 mg daily for 2 months; may be repeated if necessary after at least 2 months. For treatment and prevention of post-menopausal osteoporosis, 5 mg/daily or 35 mg/weekly. • **Zoledronic acid**: for Paget's disease, 5 mg IV as a single dose over ≥15 minutes (at least 500 mg elemental calcium twice daily (with vitamin D) for at least 10 days is recommended). For osteoporosis (in men and post-menopausal women), 5 mg IV over ≥15 minutes once a year (before first infusion give 50 000–125 000 units of vitamin D). For fracture prevention in osteopenia, 5 mg IV as a single dose every 18 months.
Route	Oral and IV.

Table 5.3.2: Selective oestrogen receptor modulators (raloxifene)	
Indications	**Post-menopausal osteoporosis**. However, it has weak potency, and its use is decreasing because more effective alternatives are preferred.
Mechanism of action	Raloxifene is a **partial oestrogen receptor agonist**. Since oestrogen inhibits osteoclasts, **raloxifene inhibits osteoclast functioning** and as a result inhibits bone resorption. It is particularly effective in **preventing vertebral fractures**.
Side-effects	Hot flushes (vasodilatation), leg cramps, peripheral oedema, influenza-like symptoms; less commonly venous thromboembolism (VTE), thrombophlebitis; rarely rashes, GI disturbances, hypertension, arterial thromboembolism, headache, breast discomfort and thrombocytopenia.
Contraindications	Breast and endometrial cancer, history of VTE, coagulopathies, cholestasis or renal impairment (severe), breastfeeding and pregnancy, and when risk factors for stroke or VTE.
Dose	60 mg/daily
Route	Oral

Table 5.3.3: Recombinant parathyroid peptide analogue (teriparatide and abaloparatide)	
Indications	Indicated for severe osteoporosis or for women who are intolerant of, or fail to respond to bisphosphonates. Abolaparatide can be initiated in patients at high risk of fracture (even before fracture has occurred).
Mechanism of action	**Teriparatide and abaloparatide stimulate osteoblast function by binding to parathyroid type 1 receptors**, ↑ calcium absorption, and ↑ renal tubular reabsorption of calcium. These effects result in **↑ bone mineral density**, **bone mass and strength**.
Side-effects	GI disorders (nausea and reflux), palpitations, dyspnoea, headache, fatigue, asthenia (weakness), depression, dizziness, vertigo, anaemia, increased sweating, muscle cramps, hypercalcaemia, injection-site reactions, sciatica, arrhythmias, insomnia, hyperuricaemia, hypertension, hypercalciuria; rarely oedema, renal impairment, postural hypotension.
Contraindications	Pre-existing hypercalcaemia, skeletal malignancies or bone metastases, metabolic bone diseases (including Paget's disease and hyperparathyroidism), unexplained raised ALP, previous radiation therapy to the skeleton, pregnancy, breastfeeding, and severe renal impairment.
Dose	Teraparatide – 20 micrograms daily (max. duration of treatment 24 months, course not to be repeated). Abaloparatide – 80 micrograms once daily (max. duration of treatment 18 months).
Monitoring	Blood pressure, ECG before initiation, and cardiac status
Route	SC

Table 5.3.4: Monoclonal antibodies (denosumab, romosozumab)	
Indications	**Osteoporosis** (for those who are unable to comply with the special instructions for administering bisphosphonates, or have intolerance / contraindications) at an increased risk of fracture or **bone metastases**.
Mechanism of action	Denosumab is a **human monoclonal antibody** that binds the cytokine **RANK-L** (receptor activator of NFκB ligand), an essential factor initiating bone turnover. **RANK-L inhibition blocks osteoclast maturation**, **function and survival**, **thus reducing bone resorption**. Romosozumab is a humanised monoclonal antibody. It binds to sclerostin (secreted by osteoblasts), preventing it from inhibiting new bone formation through the Wnt pathway. It also inhibits RANK-L which increases dependently on sclerostin.
Side-effects	Diarrhoea, constipation, infection, pain in extremity, sciatica, hypocalcaemia (fatal cases reported), hypophosphataemia, muscle spasms, hypersensitivity; less commonly cellulitis, MI, stroke, hypocalcaemia; rarely osteonecrosis of the jaw, atypical femoral fractures, osteonecrosis of the external auditory canal. After stopping there is increased risk of hypercalcaemia and vertebral fractures.

Table 5.3.4: **Monoclonal antibodies** (denosumab, romosozumab) *(continued)*	
Contraindications	Renal impairment, hypocalcaemia, previous MI or stroke, pregnancy and breastfeeding.
Dose	For osteoporosis (denosumab): 60 mg/6 months, supplement with calcium and vit D. For osteoporosis (romosozumab): 210 mg once a month for one year, supplement with calcium and vit D.
Route	SC

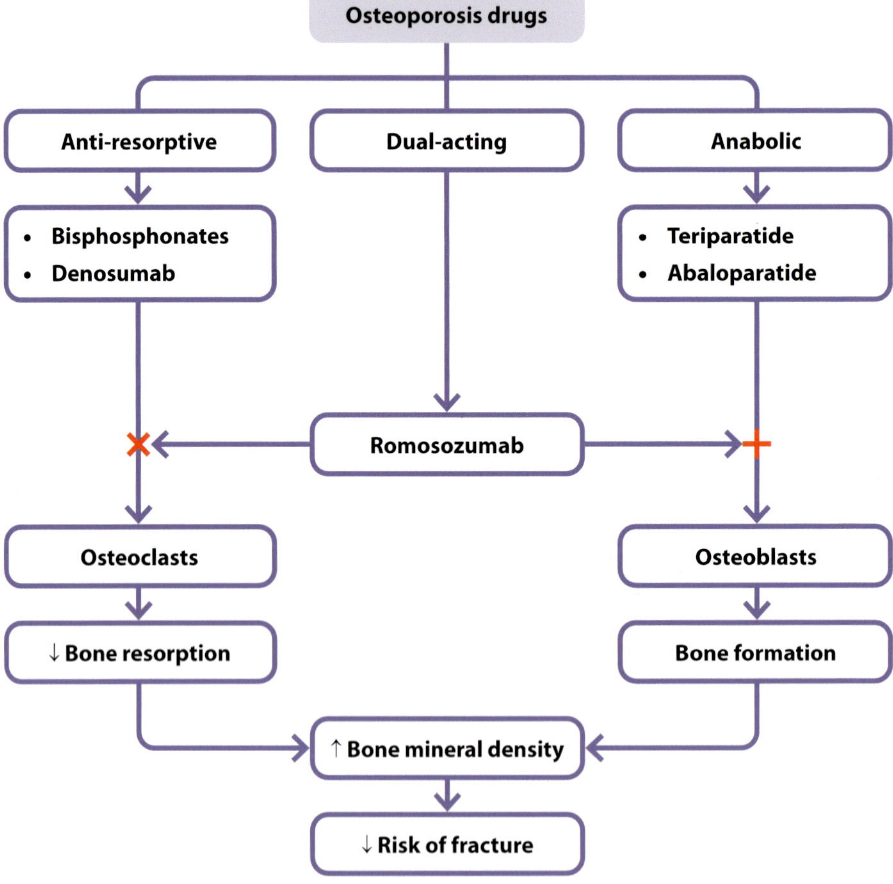

Fig. 5.3.1: Overview of the mechanism of actions of osteoporotic drugs.

5.4 DMARDs and biological agents

- **Disease-modifying antirheumatic drugs (DMARDs)** are a class of drugs commonly used to slow the disease progression of **inflammatory arthritides** such as **RA**, **AS**, **PsA**, and **SLE**.
- DMARDs fall into 3 categories, cDMARDs (conventional), bDMARDs (biologic), and tsDMARDs (targeted synthetic).
- DMARDs improve and control symptoms whilst also **delaying progression of disease** and **improving** the **extra-articular manifestations**.
- cDMARDs, such as **methotrexate**, **sulfasalazine** or **hydroxychloroquine**, are typically first-line (methotrexate is preferred unless contraindicated). Once RA has been diagnosed, cDMARDs should be started.
- **Azathioprine**, **ciclosporin**, **leflunomide** and **mycophenolate mofetil** can be used if the above fail to control disease activity. **Combination therapy** of cDMARDs are usually more effective than monotherapy.
- **Bone marrow suppression**, **liver** and **renal toxicity** are the commonest side-effects of DMARDs and therefore **FBC**, **LFTs**, and **U & Es** should be monitored regularly.
- **Biological agents** are used to treat moderate–severe RA that has not responded well to combination therapy with cDMARDs.
- In contrast to cDMARDs, biological agents are variants of the **endogenous proteins** of the immune system (usually **antibodies**).
- Examples of biological agents include **anti-TNF therapy**, **rituximab**, **tocilizumab** and other cytokine modulators (mainly interleukins).
- Biological agents are usually administered parenterally, therefore the onset of action is rapid. cDMARDs have a slow onset of action, so short-term bridging with a corticosteroid is often needed.
- **Inflammatory markers** such as **CRP** should be monitored regularly to evaluate efficacy.
- tsDMARDs include Janus kinase inhibitors (JAKi) which are selective for different combinations of JAK1,2,3, and TYK2. These enzymes are part of the JAK-STAT pathway which are used by cytokine receptors for downstream responses and gene expression.

DMARDs

Table 5.4.1: Methotrexate

Indications	**Inflammatory arthritis**, **connective tissue disease**, **vasculitis**, **GCA** and **PMR**.
Mechanism of action	• Inhibition of enzymes involved in purine metabolism, leading to accumulation of **adenosine**. Adenosine interacts with receptors on inflammatory and immune cells to regulate their function. This leads to its anti-inflammatory action. • Methotrexate causes **inhibition of T-cell activation** and suppression of intercellular adhesion molecule expression by T-cells. • Methotrexate is **anti-folate** (inhibits **dihydrofolate reductase**) and other enzymes responsible for nucleotide synthesis, but this is unlikely to contribute to its mechanism of action in RA.
Side-effects	Bone marrow suppression, GI upset (mouth ulcers), hepatotoxicity (cirrhosis) and nephrotoxicity, acute pneumonitis, pulmonary fibrosis or pulmonary oedema, hypersensitivity reactions, increased risk of infection, diarrhoea, vomiting, headache, fatigue; *uncommonly*, alopecia, arthralgia, cystitis, chills, diabetes mellitus, haemorrhage, severe cutaneous adverse reactions (SCARs), vertigo; *rarely*, asthma, brain oedema, embolism, gynaecomastia, muscle weakness, pancreatitis, psychosis, vision disorders, sexual dysfunction and vulvovaginal disorders.
Contraindications	Bone marrow dysfunction, active infections, immunosuppressed patients, GI dysfunction, severe hepatic or renal impairment, **pregnancy** (highly teratogenic – requires pre-conception counselling), breastfeeding, patients with ascites or pleural effusions.
Dose	**7.5 mg/weekly**. Adjusted according to response; max. weekly dose 25 mg.
Route	Oral, SC, IM
Pre-treatment screening and monitoring requirements	• Pre-treatment: exclude pregnancy, FBC, U & Es, LFT. • Monitoring: FBC, U & Es, LFT every 1–2 weeks until therapy has stabilized. • Report all symptoms of infection.

Table 5.4.2: Sulfasalazine	
Indications	**Inflammatory arthritides.**
Mechanisms of action	• Sulfasalazine is a combination of **5-aminosalicylic acid (5-ASA)** and **sulfapyridine**. • Its mechanism of action is not entirely understood but it is thought to inhibit NF-kB and therefore suppress responsive pro-inflammatory genes including TNF-α, inhibiting osteoclast formation via suppression on RANK-L, accumulating adenosine stimulating anti-inflammation, inhibiting the function of B-cells (but not T-cells) and suppressing IgM and IgG, and **inhibits the production of IL-8**.
Side-effects	GI upset (nausea, abdominal pain and vomiting), myelosuppression, hepatitis, rash, urine discoloration, insomnia, tinnitus; *uncommonly*, facial oedema, seizure, vasculitis and reversible hypospermia. If blood disorder occurs (first 3–6 months of treatment) then discontinue.
Cautions	Renal and hepatic hypersensitivity (contraindicated), G6PD deficiency, allergy, history of asthma, porphyria and toddlers (<2 years of age), requires folate supplementation in pregnancy.
Screening	Renal function.
Monitoring	Renal function (yearly), FBC and U & Es and LFT (monthly for first 3 months).
Dose	Initially 500 mg/24 hours, increased by 500 mg at intervals of 1 week to a max. of 2–3 g daily in divided doses. Enteric coated tablets preferred.
Route	Oral

Table 5.4.3: Hydroxychloroquine	
Indications	**RA** and **SLE**.
Mechanism of action	Likely to interfere with the **antigen presentation of B-cells** and **macrophages** by affecting the assembly of **MHC class 2 molecules**.
Side-effects	Visual changes, retinal damage, diarrhoea, headache, mood alterations, myelosuppression and skin reactions (rashes, pruritus); ECG changes, convulsions, keratopathy, ototoxicity and hair loss; *uncommonly*, anxiety, dizziness, neuromuscular dysfunction, seizure.
Cautions	Hepatic or renal impairment, epilepsy, myasthenia gravis, psoriasis, porphyria, pregnancy, breastfeeding and elderly.
Dose	200–400 mg daily
Route	Oral

Table 5.4.4: Azathioprine	
Indications	**Inflammatory arthritis**, **connective tissue disease**, **vasculitis**, **GCA** and **PMR**.
Mechanism of action	Azathioprine is cleaved to **6-mercaptopurine (6-MP)**. 6-MP functions as an **anti-metabolite** to decrease **DNA** and **RNA synthesis**, therefore causing **immunosuppression** and purine synthesis inhibition.
Side-effects	Dose-related bone marrow suppression, hypersensitivity reactions, liver impairment, cholestatic jaundice, hair loss, increased susceptibility to infections and colitis in patients also receiving corticosteroids; nausea, leucopenia, thrombocytopenia; *rarely*, SCARs, pneumonitis and neoplasms.
Contraindications	Hypersensitivity, breastfeeding, hepatic or renal impairment, pregnancy, elderly and those who have deficiency in thiopurine methyltransferase (TPMT), the enzyme which eliminates 6-MP.
Dose	1–2.5 mg/kg daily
Route	Oral

Table 5.4.5: Ciclosporin	
Indications	**RA** and **seronegative spondyloarthritis**.
Mechanism of action	• Ciclosporin **inhibits early activation of helper T-cells ($CD4^+$)** by **inhibition of the cytokine IL-2**. • Ciclosporin binds to **cyclophilin protein** and the complex then inhibits **calcineurin**, a calcium-dependent enzyme that is important in the regulation of **IL-2 production** by **helper T-cells**.
Side-effects	Nephrotoxic, hypertension, hyperlipidaemia, GI upset, hypertrichosis, gingival hyperplasia, fatigue, fever, electrolyte imbalance, hair changes, hepatic disorders, hyperglycaemia, hyperuricaemia, leucopenia, nausea, paraesthesia, renal impairments, peptic ulcer, tremor; *uncommonly*, anaemia, encephalopathy, oedema; *rarely*, gynaecomastia, idiopathic intracranial hypertension (IIH), menstrual disorder, neuropathy and myopathy.
Contraindications	Porphyria, malignant or refractory hypertension, malignancy, uncontrolled infections, hepatic or renal impairment, pregnancy and breastfeeding.
Monitoring	Monitor renal function in elderly, monitor neurological status in Behçet's syndrome.
Dose	Initially 1.5 mg/kg twice daily; this can be increased to 2.5 mg/kg twice daily after 6 weeks. Lowest possible dose should be titrated for maintenance.
Route	Oral

Table 5.4.6: Leflunomide

Indications	**RA, PsA**
Mechanism of action	• Leflunomide is a prodrug that is converted to teriflunomide. This inhibits dihydroorotate dehydrogenase which inhibits **pyrimidine nucleotide synthesis** (and therefore **DNA synthesis**) in **lymphocytes**. • It also inhibits NFκB, preventing the expression of pro-inflammatory genes.
Side-effects	GI upset (nausea, vomiting, diarrhoea and weight loss), respiratory infections, hypertension, headaches, tenosynovitis, alopecia and rash.
Contraindications	Severe immunodeficiency, severe hypoproteinaemia, significant anaemia, impaired bone marrow function, severe thrombocytopenia or leucocytopenia, serious infection, hepatic or renal impairment, pregnancy and breastfeeding, women of childbearing age (unless contraception used – it is teratogenic).
Dose	Initially 100 mg/24 hours for 3 days, then 10–20 mg/24 hours
Route	Oral

Table 5.4.7: Mycophenolate mofetil

Indications	**RA**
Mechanism of action	• Mycophenolate is a prodrug derived from the fungus ***Penicillium***. • It inhibits the enzyme **inosine monophosphate dehydrogenase** which is required for **guanosine synthesis**. • It impairs **B- and T-cell proliferation** but spares other rapidly dividing cells (because of the presence of guanosine salvage pathways in other cells).
Side-effects	GI upset (nausea, vomiting, mouth ulcers and weight loss), reversible taste loss, proteinuria and bone marrow suppression.
Contraindications	SLE, hepatic or renal impairment, nephrotoxic medications or gold therapy, pregnancy and allergy to penicillin.
Monitoring	FBC, LFT, renal profile.
Dose	1–1.5 g twice daily
Route	Oral

Biological agents

Table 5.4.8: Anti-TNF therapy	
Examples	**Infliximab**, **etanercept** and **adalimumab**.
Indications	**RA**, **AS** and **PsA**.
Mechanism of action	The pro-inflammatory cytokine TNF-α plays a key role in the pathogenesis of inflammatory arthritis by activating NFκB, proteases and protein kinases. The biological effects of TNF include activation of macrophages, T-cells and B-cells, pro-inflammatory cytokine production (IL-1, IL-6), chemokine production (IL-8, RANTES), expression of adhesion molecule (ICAM-1, E-selectin), inhibition of regulatory T-cells, RANK-L expression upregulation, matrix metalloproteinase production and induction of apoptosis. Blocking the effects of TNF-α results in **reduced inflammation within the joint, reduced angiogenesis** and **reduced joint destruction**. All anti-TNF treatments are more effective if given in **combination** with **methotrexate**. Commonly, anti-TNF therapy works by binding to TNF-α. This may result in apoptosis.
Side-effects	GI upset (constipation, diarrhoea, dyspepsia, haemorrhage, GORD), headaches, transaminitis (usually mild), upper respiratory tract infections, sinusitis, cough, renal impairment, hypotension, myocardial or cerebral ischaemia, VTE, rash, fever, seizures, lymphadenopathy and ↑ malignancy risk. Major side-effects include serious infections, congestive heart failure, drug-induced lupus and demyelinating disorders.
Contraindications	Severe acute infection, immunocompromised, herpes zoster, **possibility of TB**, heart failure, history or development of malignancy, demyelinating disorders, pregnancy (teratogenic) and breastfeeding.
Dose	See *BNF*
Route	IV and SC

Table 5.4.9: Anti-lymphocyte monoclonal antibodies (rituximab)	
Indications	**RA** and Wegener's granulomatosis.
Mechanism of action	Rituximab binds specifically to a **unique cell-surface marker CD20**, which is found on a subset of **B-cells**. B-cells have an important role in RA pathogenesis and **rituximab causes B-cell depletion**, via activation of **complement-mediated B-cell lysis**, initiation of **cell-mediated cytotoxicity via macrophages** and **induction of B-cell apoptosis**.
Side-effects	Infusion reaction, infections, haematologic adverse effects, dyspepsia, hypertension, hypotension, rhinitis, sore throat, asthenia, paraesthesia, migraine, arthralgia, muscle spasm, renal failure, tachycardia, supraventricular arrhythmias, GI effects, and urticaria, pruritus, and alopecia.
Contraindications	CVD, severe infections, pregnancy and breastfeeding.
Dose	**1 g, repeated 2 weeks after initial infusion** (in combination with methotrexate)
Route	IV

Table 5.4.10: IL-6 receptor inhibitors (tocilizumab)	
Indications	**RA**, **JRA** and **GCA**.
Mechanism of action	Tocilizumab is a **novel monoclonal antibody** that competitively **inhibits the binding of IL-6 to its receptor** (IL-6R), thereby **inhibiting the action of elevated levels of IL-6 inflammation (activation of T-cells and B-cell differentiation)**, **synovial pannus formation**, and therefore **joint destruction**.
Side-effects	GI (abdominal pain, mouth ulceration, gastritis, raised hepatic transaminases), dizziness, peripheral oedema, hypertension, hypercholesterolaemia, headache, infection, antibody formation, hypersensitivity, leucopenia, neutropenia, rash and pruritus.
Contraindications	Severe active infection, neutropenia, hepatic or renal impairment, pregnancy and breastfeeding. Caution required when history of intestinal ulceration, low absolute neutrophil count or low platelet count.
Dose	• RA: 8 mg/kg/4 weeks • JRA: see *BNF* for children • GCA: 162 mg weekly
Route	IV

Table 5.4.11: IL-17 inhibitors (secukinumab)

Indications	**AxSpA, PsA**
Mechanism of action	Secukinumab targets IL-17A, preventing it binding with the receptor. This prevents chemokine secretions and prevents the 'amplification effect' that occurs when IL-17 interacts with cytokines such as TNF-α.
Side-effects	IBD and exacerbation of Crohn's, urticaria, headache, pruritus, hypertension, arthralgia, cough, infections, malignancies, neutropenia and injection site reactions.
Contraindications	Severe active infections, TB, hepatitis B and C, HIV, hypersensitivity, demyelinating disease, optic neuritis, MS, heart failure, fever, pregnancy and breastfeeding.
Dose	150 mg every week for 5 doses. Maintenance is 150 mg every month; this can be increased up to 300 mg according to response.
Screening	FBC, LFT, U & Es, hepatitis and HIV, CXR.
Monitoring	FBC, LFT, U & Es, electrolytes after 3 months then every 6 months following.
Route	SC

Table 5.4.12: IL-23 inhibitors (guselkumab)

Indications	**PsA**
Mechanism of action	Guselkumab is a human monoclonal antibody that inhibits IL-23 by binding to the p19 subunit. This prevents IL-23 interacting with its receptor. This stops the release of chiefly IL-17 and other chemokines and cytokines.
Side-effects	Arthralgia, diarrhoea, headache, risk of infection; *uncommonly*, skin reactions.
Contraindications	Severe active infections, pregnancy and breastfeeding.
Dose	Initially 100 mg, then 100 mg after 4 weeks, then maintenance 100 mg every 8 weeks.
Screening	TB
Monitoring	Signs and symptoms of TB.
Route	SC

Table 5.4.13: JAK inhibitors (baricitinib and upadacitinib)	
Indications	**RA, AxSpA**
Mechanism of action	Baricitinib is a reversible inhibitor of JAK1 and 2. This prevents the transcription of many genes which code for inflammatory mediators. Baricitinib also modulates the signalling pathway of various interleukin, interferons and growth factors and reduces CRP levels. Upadacitinib is an ATP competitive JAK inhibitor. It affects JAK1 and 3, being more potent for the former.
Side-effects	VTE, diverticulitis, malignancy, cerebrovascular events (CVE), abdominal pain, dyslipidaemia, headache, nausea, thrombocytosis, DVT, pulmonary embolism (PE), sepsis, neoplasms, weight increase and facial swelling.
Contraindications	Severe active infections, pregnancy and breastfeeding, liver failure, renal failure, TB, low absolute lymphocyte count, low neutrophil count, severe anaemia; caution where cardiovascular, malignancy, thrombotic event and viral reactivation risk.
Dose	*Baricitinib* • Adult: 4 mg once daily, a reduced dose of 2 mg once daily is recommended for patients with certain risk factors • Elderly: 2 mg once daily *Upadacitinib* • 15 mg once daily
Screening	TB, viral hepatitis
Monitoring	Signs and symptoms of TB, periodic skin examination, haematological abnormalities, lipid profile (at 12 weeks), FBC and LFTs
Route	Oral

DO:	DO NOT:
• Monitor DMARD toxicity using the following: **bloods** (FBC, U & Es, LFTs), **urinalysis**, **BP** and **eye examination** (**for hydroxychloroquine**). • A **baseline CXR** when prescribing **methotrexate** or **anti-TNF** therapy, to rule out **pulmonary fibrosis** and **TB** respectively. • Give **folic acid** with methotrexate to reduce side-effects. • Consider performing the **TPMT test** before prescribing azathioprine.	• Prescribe methotrexate daily – a common pitfall in prescribing ('**M** is for **M**ethotrexate is for **M**onday').

Chapter 6

OSCEs

6.1	History taking	150
6.2	Examination	153
6.3	Differential diagnosis	158

6.1 History taking

This section is designed to give a brief guideline on how to take a structured history in patients with a suspected rheumatological condition.

- It is important to have a reason behind every question you ask the patient!
- There are three reasons why you would ask a question:

1. **Formulating a diagnosis**
2. **Assessing severity**
3. **Planning investigations and management**

Presenting complaint: ('Socrates')

- **Site**: see *Sec. 6.3*.
- **Onset**: *"How did it start?"*
  - Sudden onset indicates acute pathology such as **septic arthritis**, **reactive arthritis**, acute **gout or CPPD**.
  - Slow and progressive onset indicates **inflammatory arthropathy** (days / weeks) or **degenerative arthritis** (months / years).
- **Character**: *"Can you describe the pain to me?"*
- **Radiation**: *"Does the pain move anywhere else?"*
- **Association**: *"Did you notice anything else?"*
  - Pain in another joint (**additive pattern**) is associated with RA.
  - **Swelling** is associated with RA, gout / CPPD, psoriatic arthritis and other inflammatory arthritides.
  - **Redness** can be caused by septic arthritis (redness over a single joint), gout and pseudogout. RA does not cause redness of the joint.
  - **Extra-articular features** such as dry eyes in Sjögren's syndrome (see *Table 6.1.1*).
  - Feeling constantly tired and unwell may be suggestive of fibromyalgia.
  - **Fever** indicates infection, e.g. septic arthritis, or an underlying systemic inflammatory condition, e.g. SLE.
  - **Weight loss** can occur in RA, PMR and malignancy.
- **Timing**: *"When does it occur?" "How long does it last?" "How has it changed over time?"*
  - Worse on movement indicates OA.
  - Early morning stiffness which eases with movement indicates RA or AS.
- **Exacerbating / relieving factors**: *"Is there anything that makes it worse / better?"*
  - Relieved by exercise / movement → RA and AS.
  - Pain is worse on movement → OA.
- **Severity**: *"From 1 to 10, 10 being the worst pain you've ever felt, how severe is it?" "How is it affecting your life?" "Does it wake you up at night?"*

Explore activities of daily living. Good screening questions are:

- *"Can you dress yourself completely without difficulty?"*
- *"Can you walk up and down the stairs without any difficulty?"*
- Explore leisure activities and assess the patient's mood.
- Explore occupational activities.

Table 6.1.1: Extra-articular features of rheumatological disorders

Dry eyes	Sjögren's syndrome
Dry mouth	Sjögren's syndrome
Mucocutaneous ulcers	Connective tissue disorders, reactive arthritis and Behçet's disease
Dysphagia	Scleroderma
Headache	GCA
Dyspnoea	DMARDs, interstitial lung diseases secondary to RA, scleroderma or other autoimmune conditions
Photosensitivity	SLE
Fatigue	Long-standing inflammatory and autoimmune conditions
Abdominal pain	Enteropathic spondyloarthropathy (associated with Crohn's and ulcerative colitis disease)
Diarrhoea	Enteropathic spondyloarthropathy (associated with Crohn's and ulcerative colitis disease)

Past medical history

- **Osteoporosis**: any previous fractures?
- **Psoriasis** for psoriatic arthritis.
- **Mouth ulcers or recurrent skin eruption** for connective tissue disorders.
- **Uveitis** for seronegative spondyloarthropathy.
- **Previous recent infections** (upper respiratory, GI and GU infections) for reactive arthritis.
- **Peptic ulcer** when considering NSAIDs.

Drug history and allergies

- Current medication including over-the-counter medication (see *Table 6.1.2*).
- Any drug allergies? If so, what happens when patient develops the allergy?

Table 6.1.2: Specific drugs associated with rheumatological disorders

Steroids	Can cause glucocorticoid-induced osteoporosis. Other side-effects should also be monitored (see *Chapter 5*)
Diuretics	Can cause gout
Minocycline, isoniazid, terbinafine, phenytoin, carbamazepine and sulfasalazine	Can cause drug-induced lupus

Family history

- Ask about any conditions that run in the family, specifically rheumatological conditions such as RA, SLE, AS and nodal OA.
- If there is any family history, ask about the age of onset and prognosis.

Social history

- **Ask about alcohol consumption and smoking:**
  - Alcohol intake is a risk factor for gout.
  - Smoking is a risk factor for osteoporosis.
- **Ask about occupation:**
  - Physical stress on joints can lead to degenerative arthritis (e.g. carpenter – OA of the hand; plumber/roofer – OA of the knee).
- **Explore the patient's social status:**
  - Ask about marriage status, family support and living accommodation.
  - Ask about impact of symptoms on their activities of daily living.
  - If the patient is living in two-storey accommodation and has poor mobility, referral to an occupational therapist to assess the situation at the patient's home (holistic approach) may be required.

ICE: ideas, concerns and expectations

- *"Do you have any thoughts as to what might be happening?"*
- *"Is there anything in particular which is concerning you?"*
- *"What were you hoping we could do for you?"*

6.2 Examination

This section will cover a useful screening examination known as the GALS: gait, arms, legs and spine. Examination of the hands and wrists will be covered in more detail at the end of the section, since it is a common presentation in rheumatology. Some useful videos on musculoskeletal examination are to be found at bit.ly/VA-MSK.

The GALS screening examination

Before starting the examination, wash your hands, introduce yourself, explain what you are going to do and obtain consent from the patient. Ensure that the patient is adequately exposed. There are three screening questions that form part of the examination:

1. *"Do you have any pain or stiffness in your muscle joints or back?"*
2. *"Can you dress yourself completely without any difficulties?"*
3. *"Can you walk up and down the stairs without any difficulties?"*

Gait

Ask the patient to walk and look for the following:

- Phases of gait: heel strike, stance, push-off and swing
- Loss of symmetry
- Antalgic (painful) gait
- Use of walking aids
- Difficulty with transfer (sitting and standing from a chair).

Arms

- **Look**
    - Skin: discoloration, nodules, nail signs: **pitting**, **onycholysis** and **hyperkeratosis** all suggest psoriatic arthritis.
    - Muscles: muscle wasting or hypertrophy.
    - Joints: swelling and erythema.
- **Feel**
    - Skin temperature: if skin is warm, this indicates active inflammation or infection.
    - Joint swelling: bony swelling indicates degenerative arthritis; rubbery swelling indicates inflammatory arthritis.
    - Pain on squeezing the MCP joints suggests RA.
- **Move**
    - Assess pronation and supination of the hands by asking the patient to face their palms downwards and upwards, respectively, while elbows are held at the side of their abdomen to exclude any shoulder movement (*Fig. 6.2.1a*).
    - Assess the power grip of each hand by asking the patient to squeeze your finger. Assess pinch grip precision and strength by trying to break the patient's pinch.

- Ask the patient to flex and extend their wrist, elbow and shoulder.
- Assess shoulder adduction and internal rotation by asking the patient to place their hands behind their back as high as they can (*Fig. 6.2.1b*).
- Assess shoulder external rotation and abduction by asking the patient to place their hands behind their head with elbows as far back as possible (*Fig. 6.2.1c*).

Note: When examining the joint movements, look for any discomfort / pain or restrictions.

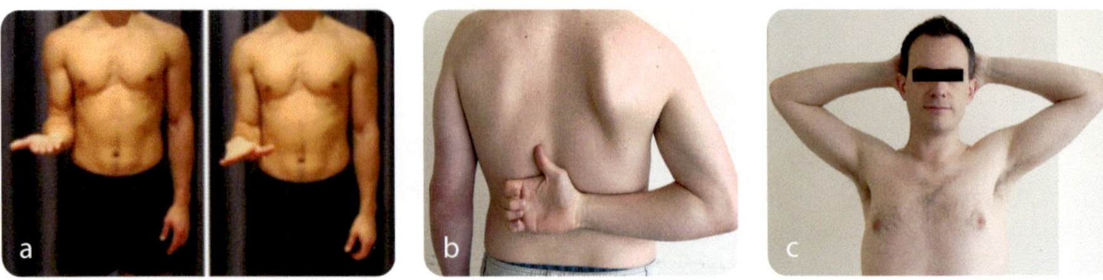

Fig. 6.2.1: **(a)** Supination and pronation of the hand; **(b)** shoulder adduction and internal rotation; **(c)** shoulder abduction and external rotation.

Legs

For examination of the legs, the patient should be lying down on a couch.

- **Look**
  - Skin: discoloration, nodules, callosity (thickening of skin, often on the sole of the foot).
  - Muscles: wasting and fasciculation.
  - Joints: swelling, asymmetry and deformity.
- **Feel**
  - Skin: for temperature.
  - Joints: for tenderness (especially along the knee joint margins), warmth and swelling.
- **Move**
  - Ask the patient to bend each knee in turn.
  - Flex and extend the patient's knee with one hand while placing the other hand on the knee joint, in order to feel for any crepitus (*Fig. 6.2.2*).

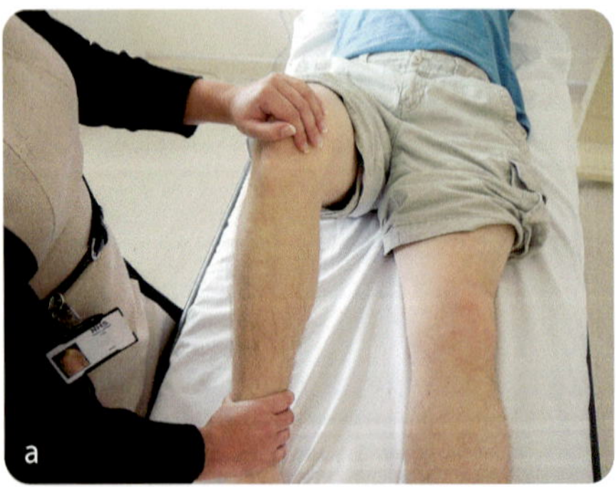

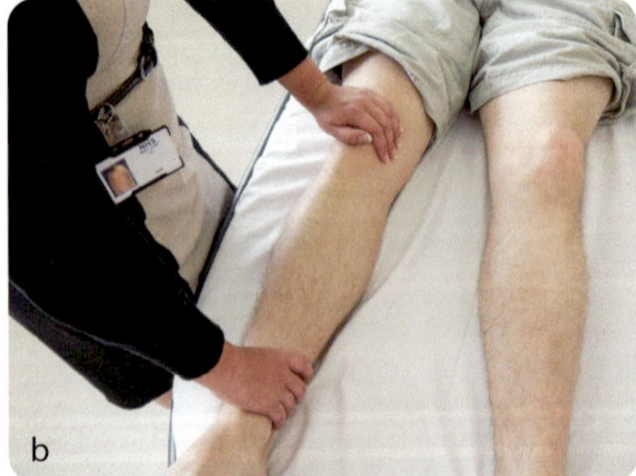

Fig. 6.2.2: Feeling for any knee crepitus while passively flexing **(a)** and extending **(b)** the knee.

- Hold the knee and hip at 90 degrees of flexion and rotate the hip internally and externally (*Fig. 6.2.3*). Keep an eye on the patient's face to elicit any pain or discomfort.

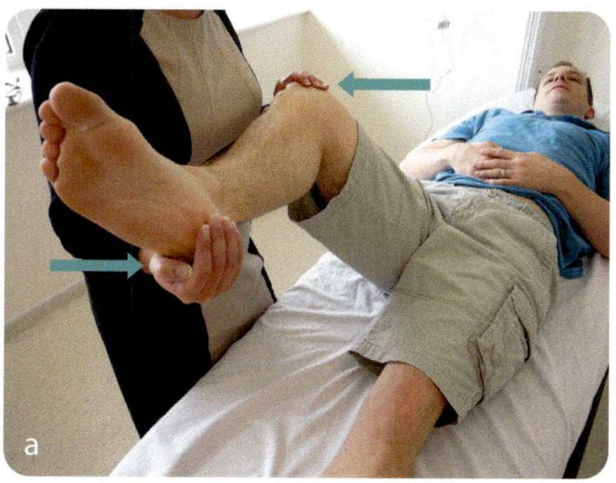

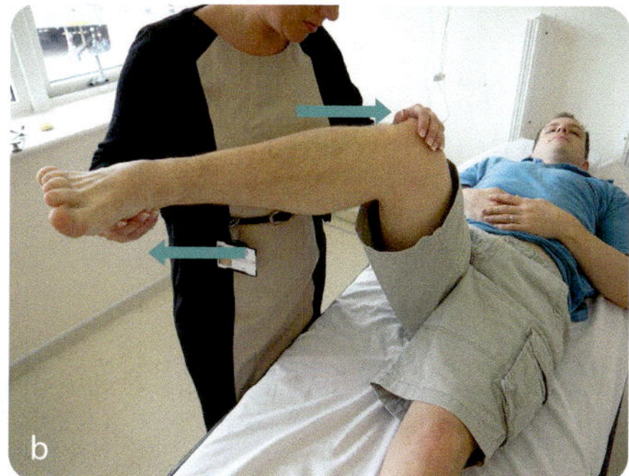

Fig. 6.2.3: **(a)** External rotation of the hip; **(b)** internal rotation of the hip.

Spine

- **Look**
  - Look from the front.
  - Look from the back for normal muscle bulk, to see whether the spine is straight or if there is scoliosis (lateral deviation of the spine).
  - Look from the side for normal cervical lordosis, thoracic kyphosis and lumbar lordosis. Also, look for abnormal kyphosis and fixed flexion deformity.
- **Feel**
  - Feel for any tenderness along the vertebral bodies.
- **Move**
  - Ask the patient to put their ear on their shoulder to elicit lateral flexion of the neck.
  - Ask the patient to flex and extend their neck to elicit normal flexion and extension of the neck.
  - Ask the patient to touch their toes to elicit normal flexion of the lumbar spine.
  - Ask the patient to turn their body on either side to elicit spinal rotation.

Hand and wrist examination

Before examination

Before starting the examination, wash your hands, introduce yourself, explain what you are going to do and obtain consent from the patient. Ensure that the patient's hand, wrist and elbows are exposed adequately.

Look

Start with dorsum then move to the palm and look for any abnormalities, noting whether they are symmetrical or asymmetrical.

- **Nails**
    - Psoriatic changes: pitting, onycholysis, subungual hyperkeratosis.
    - Nail fold vasculitis.
- **Skin**
    - Any scars (e.g. previous carpal tunnel release surgery).
    - Palmar erythema (RA).
    - Bruising and thinning (long-term steroid use).
    - Rheumatoid nodules (especially around the elbows in RA).
- **Joints**
    - Bouchard's nodes (PIP joints) and Heberden's nodes (DIP joints) in OA.
    - Swelling of the MCP joints (RA).
    - Ulnar deviation, swan neck deformity and boutonnière deformity in RA.
- **Muscles and tendons**
    - Look for muscle wasting in thenar and hypothenar prominences of the hand (to elicit nerve damage).
    - Look for prominent extrinsic flexor tendons on the ulnar aspect of the hand (Dupuytren's contracture).

Feel

- Always ask if the patient is in any pain before touching their hands.
- Feel for temperature over the forearm, wrist and MCP joints on both sides.
- Feel for the muscle bulk and any tendon thickening (Dupuytren's contracture).
- Assess nerve sensation by touching the hypothenar (ulnar nerve) and thenar (median nerve) eminences and the dorsal side over the thumb and index, as well as the web space (radial nerve).
- Feel for peripheral pulses.
- Gently squeeze over the MCP joints while watching the patient's face to elicit any pain.
- **Bimanually palpate** any MCP joints that appear to be swollen or tender with the thumbs above and index finger below the MCP joint.
- Both PIP and wrist joints should be palpated in a similar manner.
- Feel the elbow along the ulnar border for any nodules.

Move

- Movement is examined actively and passively.
- Look for limitation of the normal range.
- Assessing power is recommended.

- **Wrist**
  - Flexion and extension (*Fig. 6.2.4*).
  - Ulnar and radial deviation.
  - Pronation and supination.

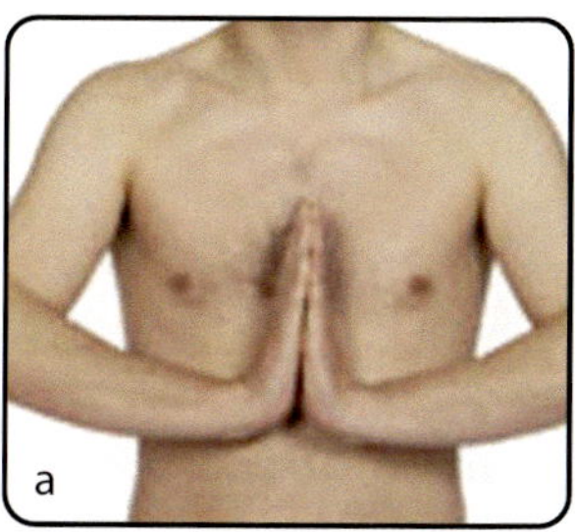

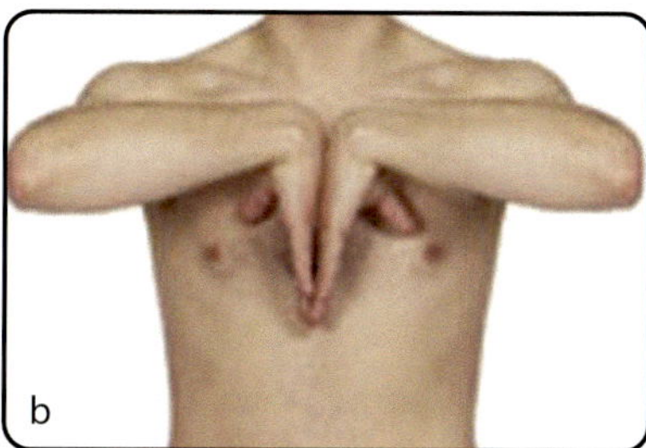

Fig. 6.2.4: **(a)** Excessive wrist extension **(b)** Excessive wrist flexion.

- **Fingers**
  - Flexion and extension: ask the patient to make a fist and open it again.
  - Abduction: ask the patient to spread their fingers out with the palm facing downwards.
  - While in the same position, assess the extensor power by pushing the fingers downwards; this specifically examines the radial nerve.
  - Also assess the power of finger abduction; this specifically examines the ulnar nerve.
- **Thumbs**
  - Flexion
  - Extension
  - Abduction
  - Adduction
  - Opposition
- **Function**
  - Assess hand grip by asking the patient to squeeze your fingers.
  - Assess pencil grip.
  - Ask them to pick up a small object (e.g. a coin).

After examination

- Consider vascular and neurological examinations of the upper limb.
- If appropriate, indicate that you would like to order some tests.
- Ensure the patient is comfortable and offer your help to put clothes back on.
- Offer differential diagnoses.

OSCE tips: Assessing hand movement

- Sometimes it is better to demonstrate movements to the patient, e.g. in elderly individuals who might find it difficult to carry out certain instructions (*"Mr Smith, can you move your thumb like this?"*).
- If the patient's joint is acutely tender, avoid passive movement.
- If there is restriction in range of movement (ROM), find out if this is mild, moderate or severe.
- Find out the cause of the restricted ROM; i.e. whether it is due to **pain or mechanical restriction**.
- Find out if the movement is **restricted passively, actively or both**.
- Pain on active or resisted movement alone indicates tendinopathies.
- When assessing the power, it is best to oppose the patient's movement with the same movement, i.e. if you are assessing index flexion power, oppose the patient's index flexion with your index flexion.

6.3 Differential diagnosis

This section will discuss the differential diagnosis of common presentations in rheumatology.

DIP and PIP joint pain

- **Osteoarthritis (OA):** common in females (usually >40 years of age) and presents with bony swellings (more commonly in DIP than PIP joints):
  - DIP: Heberden's nodes
  - PIP: Bouchard's nodes
- **Rheumatoid arthritis (RA):** presents with soft tissue swelling and tenderness that is usually symmetrical (more common in PIP than DIP joints).
- **Spondyloarthropathy** (e.g. psoriatic or reactive arthritis): presents similarly to RA; however, it is usually asymmetrical. Psoriatic arthritis may affect both PIP and DIP joints but characteristically affects the DIP joint.

Note: a more common presentation of psoriatic arthritis and reactive arthritis occur in large joints (asymmetrical and oligo-articular).

MCP soft tissue swelling and tenderness

- **RA:** a common presentation of RA, usually in both hands; tenderness can be elicited by gently squeezing the MCP joints.
- **Spondyloarthropathy:** usually presents asymmetrically with dactylitis (*Box 6.3.1*).

Box 6.3.1: Dactylitis

- Inflammation of the entire digit (either finger or toe)
- Swells up into a sausage shape and can become painful
- Causes of dactylitis include:
  - Spondyloarthropathy (common)
  - Sickle-cell anaemia (usually presents in children >4 years of age)
  - Tuberculosis (rare)
  - Sarcoidosis (rare)

Thumb base pain

- **1st carpometacarpal (CMC) in OA:** common presentation in females aged >40 with an occupational history of repetitive hand movement. Examination reveals bony swellings of the 1st CMC joint.
  - **De Quervain's tenosynovitis:** associated with chronic overuse such as in jobs or hobbies that involve repetitive hand and wrist motions.

Elbow pain

- **Lateral epicondylitis** (tennis elbow): repetitive use of the extensor muscles which are attached to the lateral epicondyle. It presents with tenderness at the lateral epicondyle, which can be exacerbated by extension of the wrist against resistance.
- **Medial epicondylitis** (golfer's elbow): repetitive use of the flexor muscles that are attached to the medial epicondyle. Presents with tenderness at the medial epicondyle, which can be exacerbated by flexion of the wrist against resistance.
- **Olecranon bursitis:** presents with local soft tissue swelling over the olecranon process. Fluctuant swelling is seen in conditions such as overuse or gout.
- **Rheumatoid nodules:** these are similar to bursitis but are **more firm** and are usually located on the ulnar side of the elbow.

Trapezius muscle pain

- Fibromyalgia: associated **widespread pain**, above and below the waist as well as the axial skeletal system, for at least **3 months**.

Thoracic spine pain

- **Ankylosing spondylitis:** usually presents in young men with limited range of movement in the lumbar spine and reduced chest expansion.
- **Osteoporotic vertebral fractures:** usually present in elderly women with dorsal kyphosis.

Lower back pain

Acute

- **Disc prolapse:** usually presents with mechanical back pain and often leads to sciatica (buttock pain and numbness or weakness shooting down the leg and foot).

Chronic

- **Fibromyalgia**.
- If the pain is associated with sciatica, rule out **spinal stenosis**.
- **Osteomalacia / hypovitaminosis D:** usually presents with pathological fractures, and bone pain and tenderness.
- **Ankylosing spondylitis:** presents with dull back pain that radiates to the hip / buttocks); usually associated with stiffness.

Hip pain

- **OA of the hip:** a common cause of chronic hip pain.
- Trochanteric bursitis: presents with lateral hip pain which is very sore to lie on.

Knee pain

Anterior

- **Chondromalacia patellae:** damage to the patella cartilage which usually presents in young individuals engaged in active sports. Pain is typically felt after prolonged sitting.
- **Pre- or infra-patellar bursitis ('housemaid's knee' or 'clergyman's knee'):** anterior swelling and tenderness; common amongst plumbers, cleaners, carpet fitters and any other people who may have to kneel a lot.

Diffuse

- **OA of the knee:** usually presents with crepitus, reduced range of movement and bony swelling (late).
- **RA of the knee:** symmetrical joint pain with swollen, warm and effused joints.
- **Ligament or meniscal injury:** sudden onset and history of recent trauma. Usually presents with locking of the knee.

Foot pain

- **Gout:** acute, asymmetrical, swollen, red joint. Always rule out septic arthritis!
- **OA of the 1st metatarso-phalangeal (MTP) joint:** chronic, bony swelling.
- **Dactylitis:** swelling of the entire toe which can be red and painful. This occurs in spondyloarthropathies.
- **RA:** symmetrical pain of the MTP joints which is accompanied by tenderness and swelling.

Appendix

Photograph acknowledgments

Please note that the following images are reproduced under the Creative Commons Attribution Share-Alike Licence; reproduced from www.wikipedia.com: Figs. 7.2.1(b) and (c), Figs. 7.2.2–7.2.4.

Fig. 2.1.1

Adapted by permission from Macmillan Publishers Ltd: *Nature Reviews Drug Discovery*, 2007; 6(1): 75–92, V. Strand *et al.*, 'Biologic therapies in rheumatology: lessons learned, future directions'.

Fig. 2.1.2 (a) Boutonnière and swan neck deformities

Reprinted from *Pathophysiology*, vol. 12, R. Khurana & S. M. Berney, 'Clinical aspects of rheumatoid arthritis', pp. 153–165, 2005, with permission from Elsevier.

Fig. 2.1.2 (a) Ulnar deformity

Reproduced from www.joint-pain-solutions.com/rheumatoid-arthritis-pictures.html

Fig. 2.1.2 (b)

Courtesy of Dr F. Gaillard, Radiopaedia.org.

Fig. 2.2.1

Adapted by permission from Macmillan Publishers Ltd: *Nature Reviews Drug Discovery*, **4:** pp. 331–344, Heike A. Wieland *et al.*, 'Osteoarthritis - an untreatable disease?' (April 2005).

Fig. 2.2.2

Reproduced from *Ann Rheum Dis* (1999) **58:** 675–678, Colin Alexander, 'Heberden's and Bouchard's nodes', with permission from BMJ Publishing Group Ltd.

Fig. 2.2.3

Reproduced from www.kneeandhip.co.uk/hip/hip-pain/hip-osteoarthritis/

Fig. 2.2.4

Reproduced from http://stemcelldoc.wordpress.com/2011/11/13/kellgren-lawrence-classification-knee-osteoarthritis-classification-and-treatment-options/

Fig. 2.2.6

Reproduced from www.kneeandhip.co.uk/arthritis/default.aspx

Fig. 2.4.1

Reproduced from http://crdq.ca/en/participants/fiches-dermatologiques/psoriatic-arthritis/9/

Fig. 2.4.2

Reproduced with kind permission from Springer Science+Business Media B.V.; *Atlas of Rheumatology* by E. Matteson *et al.*

Fig. 2.4.3

Image © Dr Soumya Chatterjee, reproduced from http://bestpractice.bmj.com/best-practice/monograph/1191/resources/image/bp/6.html

Fig. 2.4.4

Reproduced from www.windsorfoot.com/foot_achilles_problems_windsor.php

Fig. 2.4.5

Reproduced from www.sich.co.uk/hypnotherapy/hypnotherapy-for-psoriasis/

Fig. 2.4.6

Reproduced from *Ann Rheum Dis* (2005) **64:** ii58–ii60 with permission from D. McGonagle

Fig. 2.5.2

Reproduced from www.scielo.br/pdf/rb/v40n1/en_10.pdf

Fig. 2.5.3

Reproduced from www.medicalpicturesinfo.com

Fig. 2.6.2

Reproduced courtesy of Life in the Fast Lane, www.lifeinthefastlane.com

Fig. 2.6.3

Reproduced courtesy of Drs Wiesner and Kaufman, Centers for Disease Control and Prevention.

Fig. 2.7.2 (a)

Reproduced from www.flickr.com – photo by "mobiledoc".

Fig. 2.7.2 (b)

Figure reproduced with permission from Arthritis Research UK (www.arthritisresearchuk.org) from: Roddy E. *Gout: presentation and management in primary care*. Reports on the Rheumatic Diseases (Series 6), Hands On 9. Arthritis Research UK; 2011 Summer

Fig. 2.7.2 (c)

Reproduced from http://hcp.stampoutgout.co.uk/gout-clinical-features/tophi.htm

Fig. 2.8.1 (a)

Reproduced from *Ann Rheum Dis*, 'Chondrocalcinosis and Gitelman's syndrome. A new association? J. C. Cobeta-Garcia *et al.*, **57**: 748–749 (1998), with permission from BMJ Publishing Group Ltd.

Fig. 2.8.1 (b)

Reproduced from *Ann Rheum Dis*, 'European League Against Rheumatism recommendations for calcium pyrophosphate deposition. Part I: terminology and diagnosis'. W. Zhang *et al.*, **70**(4): 563–570 (2011), with permission from BMJ Publishing Group Ltd.

Fig. 2.9.1

Reproduced from *Arthritis & Rheumatism*, Jennette *et al.*, (**65**), 1–11 (2013), with permission from John Wiley & Sons.

Fig. 2.9.2

Reproduced from www.thelancetstudent.com/legacy/2010/11/16/the-lancet-seminar-antiphosholipid-syndrome/

Fig. 2.9.3

Image courtesy of a Vasculitis UK member, www.vasculitis.org.uk

Fig. 2.9.4

Reproduced from *BMJ*, 'ABC of arterial and vascular disease: Vasculitis'. C.O.S. Savage *et al.*, **320**, 2000, with permission from BMJ Publishing Group Ltd.

Fig. 2.9.5

Image courtesy of a Vasculitis UK member, www.vasculitis.org.uk

Fig. 2.9.6

Figure reproduced courtesy of Dr Yusuf Yazici.

Fig. 2.10.1
Image reproduced courtesy of Dr G. Pountain and Dr B. Hazleman.

Fig. 2.12.3
Image, showing typical clinical presentation of a malar (butterfly) rash in a 31 year old female patient with SLE, reproduced courtesy of Dr Ina Hadshiew.

Fig. 2.12.4
Image provided by a lupus patient.

Fig. 2.12.5
Reproduced from http://pimaderm.com/Conditions-Treated/Hair-and-nail-conditions

Fig. 2.12.6
Reproduced under the Open Government Licence from www.dwp.gov.uk

Fig. 2.13.2
Reproduced from The Pulse, http://clinicalexamskills.blogspot.co.uk/2010/08/dermatomyositis.html

Fig. 2.13.3
Reproduced from *BMJ*, 'Case reports: A woman with muscles pain, weakness, and macular rash'. A.G. Tristano, 2009, with permission from BMJ Publishing Group Ltd.

Fig. 2.13.4
Reproduced with permission from St John's Institute of Dermatology (King's College), London.

Fig. 2.14.1
Reproduced courtesy of Dr Alfredo Aguirre (School of Dental Medicine, University at Buffalo, The State University of New York).

Fig. 2.14.2
Reproduced from www.eyedocs.co.uk/ophthalmology-learning/articles/cornea/505-schirmers-test

Figs. 2.15.1 (b) and (d)
Reproduced with permission from: Pope J. 'Limited cutaneous systemic sclerosis'. *BMJ Best Practice*. www.bestpractice.bmj.com. Accessed 24 October 2013.

Fig. 2.15.1 (c)
Reproduced from www.raynauds.org.uk/images/stories/PDF/localised08.pdf

Fig. 2.15.1 (e)
Reproduced from www.raynauds.org.uk/raynauds/raynauds

Fig. 2.15.2
Reproduced with permission from www.sclero.org – photo by Hazel McCoy.

Fig. 2.17.2
Reproduced from www.prestonchiropractic.co.uk/doctor/chiropractor/chiropractic-Preston/chiropractic-topics/chiropractic-for-osteoporosis-pain-relief

Fig. 2.17.3
Reproduced from http://emedicalppt.blogspot.co.uk/2011/04/hip-fractures-in-elderly.html

Fig. 2.17.4
Reproduced from www.imageinterpretation.co.uk/wrist.html

Fig. 2.18.2

Reproduced courtesy of Dr C. Restrepo, The Rothman Institute.

Fig. 2.18.3

Reproduced from www.surgicalnotes.co.uk

Fig. 2.18.4

Reproduced courtesy of Dr C. Restrepo, The Rothman Institute.

Fig. 3.1.2

Reproduced with permission from www.childortho.com/deformity_hemi_epiphysiodesis.html

Fig. 3.1.3

Reproduced courtesy of Dr Frank Noyes.

Fig. 4.2.1

Images obtained from the Department of Immunology, Royal Liverpool University Hospital, with permission.

Fig. 4.3.1

Reproduced from the Rheumination blog at http://rheumination.typepad.com

Fig. 4.3.2 (a)

Reproduced from *BMJ*, 'Picture quiz: An acutely swollen knee', R. Maggio *et al.*, **340**: (2010), with permission from BMJ Publishing Group Ltd.

Fig. 4.3.2 (b)

Reproduced courtesy of Dr Ann K. Rosenthal (Medical College of Wisconsin).

Fig. 6.2.1 (a)

Reproduced from http://orthoanswer.org/hand-wrist/fracture-scaphoid/treatment.html

Figs. 6.2.1 (b) and (c); Figs. 6.2.2 and 6.2.3

Reproduced from www.osceskills.com under the terms of the Creative Commons Attribution Share-Alike Licence.

Note: We are making the following images freely available under the terms of the Creative Commons Attribution Share-Alike Licence: Figs. 2.1.3, 2.1.4, 2.5.1, the figure illustrating Schober's test, 2.12.2, 2.15.1 (a), 2.16.1, 4.1.1, 4.1.2 and 4.1.3.

Index

Bold indicates main entry

abaloparatide, 91, 135, 137, 138
ACE, 82
acromegaly, 44
adalimumab, 13, 28, 33, 108, 144
Adcal, 101
alkaline phosphatase, *see* ALP
allodynia, 73
allopurinol, 42, 45
alopecia, 63, 64, 65, 66, 135, 140, 143, 145
ALP, 93, 94, 95, 96, 101, 114, 137
amaurosis fugax, 55, 56, 57
amenorrhoea, 65, 92
amitriptyline, 87
amyloidosis, 10, 31, 76
ANA, 27, 32, 37, 62, 64, 66, 71, 75, 78, 79, 81, 104, 107, 108, 116, 118
anakinra, 13, 42
anaphylaxis, 125
aneurysm, 48, 53, 56, 123
angiotensin-converting enzyme, *see* ACE
anifrolumab, 68
ankylosing spondylitis, 24, **30–4**, 104, 159
anorexia, 21, 51
anti-cardiolipin, 64, 67, 117
anti-centromere antibody, 81, 82, 117, 119
anti-dsDNA, 62, 64, 66, 67, 116, 118
anti-IL, 13, 28, 33, 42, 46, 54, 108, 141, 142, **145–6**
anti-Jo-1, 71, 72, 117, 118, **119**
anti-La, 74, 75, 76, 117, **119**
anti-lymphocyte monoclonal antibodies, 145
anti-Mi-2, 71
anti-MPO, 53, 118
antinuclear antibody, *see* ANA
antiphospholipid syndrome, 53, 62, 64, 66, **67**, 117
anti-PR3, 53, 118
anti-RNA, 81, 82
anti-Ro, 74, 76, 117, 118, **119**
anti-Scl-70, 81, 82, 116, 118, **119**
anti-Smith, 64, 66, 118, **119**
anti-SSA, *see* anti-Ro
anti-SSB, *see* anti-La
anti-Th/To, 117, **119**
anti-TNF, 13, 28, 33, 38, 108, 139, **144**, 147
anti-topoisomerase, *see* anti-Scl-70
anxiety, 84, 85, 86, 141
apoptosis, 8, 15, 63, 93, 119, 135, 144, 145
arthralgia, 33, 50, 51, 65, 75, 76, 140, 145, 146
arthritis
  juvenile idiopathic (JIA), 103–8
  juvenile rheumatoid (JRA), *see* JIA
  mutilans, 26
  osteo-, 10, **15–19**, 41, 44, 45, 96, 158
  psoriatic, 11, 24, **25–9**, 118, 150, 151, 153, 156, 158
  reactive, 27, **35–8**, 107, 150, 151, 158
  rheumatoid, **8–14**, 16, 17, 18, 21, 22, 24, 26, 27, 29, 37, 47, 49, 60, 61, 66, 70, 74, 75, 84, 89, 90, 110, 111, 112, 113, 116, 117, 118, 119, 121, 122, 124, 125, 130, 133, 134, 139–47, 150–4, 158, 160
  septic, **20–3**, 37, 41, 45, 107, 112, 120, 121, 122, 150, 160
aspirin, 40, 67, 108
asthma, 49, 51, 52, 112, 130, 131, 140, 141
azathioprine, 54, 61, 68, 73, 111, 133, 139, **142**, 147

Baker's cysts, 11
balanitis, 36
bamboo spine, 30, 32
baricitinib, 13, 114, **147**
BASDAI, 33
Bath Ankylosing Spondylitis Disease Activity Index, *see* BASDAI
bDMARDs, *see* biological agents

Behçet's disease, 49, **51–3**, 142, 151
belimumab, 68
beta-lactams, 47
biological agents, 12, 13, 28, 33, 54, 68, 108, 114, 115, 116, 139, **144–7**
birefringence, 41, 45, 121
bisphosphonate, 58, 61, 91, 92, 96, 99, 134, **135–6**, 137, 138
blepharitis, 75
blood tests, 110–15
BMI, 19, 89, 99
body mass index, *see* BMI
Bouchard's nodes, 16, 17, 156, 158
boutonnière, 9, 156
bradycardia, 132
bursitis, 15, 22, 27, 60, 86
 infra-patellar, 160
 olecranon, 159
 pre-patellar, 160

calciferol, 102
calcineurin, 67, 142
calcinosis, 79, 80
calcitonin, 96
calcium pyrophosphate disease, *see* CPPD
c-ANCA, 47, 48, 53, 116, 118
candidiasis, 75, 76
carbamazepine, 151
cardiac, 36, 53, 68, 83, 94, 130, 137
CBT, 87, 128
cefotaxime, 22
celecoxib, 129, 130
chlamydia, 35, 37, 38
chondrocalcinosis, 44, 45, 124
chondromalacia patellae, 160
Churg–Strauss syndrome, *see* CSS
ciclosporin, 28, 40, 73, 76, 139, **142**
claustrophobia, 125
clergyman's knee, 160
cognitive behavioural therapy, *see* CBT
colchicine, 42, 45, 46
colitis, 142
 ulcerative, 134, 151
corticosteroids, 12, 13, 28, 33, 38, 42, 46, 58, 60, 76, 112, **133–4**, 139, 142
COX enzyme, 129, 130, 133
CPPD, 17, 22, **44–6**, 112, 121, 122, 150
C-reactive protein, *see* CRP
crepitus, 16, 17, 154, 160
CREST syndrome, 78, 79, 80, 81, 117, 119
Crohn's disease, 151
CRP, 11, 12, 17, 21, 22, 27, 32, 33, 37, 45, 56, 57, 58, 60, 66, 67, 71, 107, **113**, 139, 147
CSS, **47–53**, 118
cyclophosphamide, 53, 68, 83
cytomegalovirus, 79
cytotoxic, 63, 69, 145

dactylitis, 24, 26, 27, 36, 105, 158, 160
de Quervain's tenosynovitis, 158
denosumab, 91, 96, 135, **137–8**
dermatomyositis, **69–73**, 133
DEXA scan, 90, 91, 92, 123, **125**
diabetes mellitus, 21, 40, 66, 89, 101, 133, 134, 140
diarrhoea, 24, 42, 51, 65, 82, 130, 135, 137, 140, 141, 143, 144, 146, 151
diclofenac, 13, 129, 130, 131
diplopia, 55, 56
Disease Activity Score, 12, 13, 14, 33, 41
disease-modifying antirheumatic drugs, *see* DMARDs
DMARDs, 12, 13, 28, 73, 112, 113, 114, **139–47**, 151
dry eyes, 10, **74–7**, 150, 151
dry mouth, **74–7**, 132, 151
Dupuytren's contracture, 156
dysmotility, 70, 72, 79, 81
dyspareunia, 74
dyspepsia, 135, 144, 145
dysphagia, 70, 72, 74, 79, 80, 135, 151
dysphonia, 70
dysplasia, 95
dysuria, 36, 38

ECG, 64, 66, 137, 141
echocardiogram, 53, 66, 81
eGFR, 114
ENA, 116, 117, 118, **119**
encephalitis, 51, 105, 142

endocarditis, 63, 65, 117
enthesitis, 24, 26, 30, 32, 33, 36, 37, 103, 104, 106, 107
epilepsy, 141
epistaxis, 50, 54
erythema, 21, 22, 41, 45, 51, 64, 70, 153, 156
  macular, 70
  nail-fold, 70
  nodosum, 51
  palmar, 156
estimated glomerular filtration rate, *see* eGFR
extractable nuclear antigen antibodies, *see* ENA

fasciitis, 24, 36, 71
FBC, 11, 12, 32, 53, 56, 58, 66, 67, 110, 139, 140, 141, 143, 146, 147
femoral, 17, 99, 101, 137
ferritin, 11, 105, 107, 111
fibrinogen, 112, 113, 120
fibrocartilage, 30, 44
fibromyalgia, 61, **84–7**, 150, 159
flucloxacillin, 22
Fracture Risk Assessment Tool, *see* FRAX
FRAX, 90, 91
full blood count, *see* FBC

gait, 17, 102, 153
  waddling, 99, 100
  see also GALS
GALS, 153
gamma-glutamyltransferase, 114
gastro-oesophageal reflux disease, *see* GORD
GCA, **47–58**, 59, 60, 61, 113, 125, 126, 133, 134, 140, 142, 145, 151
giant cell arteritis, *see* GCA
glomerulonephritis, 48, 49, 51, 53, 114
glucocorticoids, 13, 19, 57, 58, 67, 68, 76, 88, 98, 108, 112, 125, 133, 151
glucose, 121, 122
gold therapy, 143
golimumab, 28, 33
GORD, 79, 80, 144
gout, 22, 27, 37, **39–43**, 44, 45, 112, 113, 114, 121, 122, 133, 150, 151, 152, 159, 160
granulomas, 55
granulomatosis, **47–54**, 116, 118, 145
guselkumab, 146

HAART, 98
haemarthrosis, 22, 120
haemochromatosis, 44
headache, 55, 56, 57, 58, 65, 86, 130, 136, 137, 140, 141, 143, 144, 145, 146, 147, 151
heart failure, 52, 65, 80, 134, 144, 146
Heberden's nodes, 16, 17, 156, 158
Henoch–Schönlein purpura, *see* HSP
hepatitis, 49, 50, 53, 114, 118, 119, 141, 146, 147
highly active antiretroviral treatment, *see* HAART
histamine, 47, 133
HIV, 25, 27, 35, 146
HLA, 8, 9, 24, 25, 30, 31, 32, 35, 37, 47, 59, 63, 69, 70, 74, 75, 103, 104, 105, 106, 107
HSP, 47–54
human immunodeficiency virus, *see* HIV
human leucocyte antigen, *see* HLA
hydrocortisone, 133, 134
hyperalgesia, 84, 85
hypercalcaemia, 94, 137
hypercalcinuria, 89
hyperkalaemia, 53
hyperkeratosis, 26, 153, 156
hyperplasia, 15, 25, 142
hypersensitivity, 93, 130, 133, 137, 140, 141, 142, 145, 146
hypocalcaemia, 99, 100, 135, 137, 138
hypomagnesaemia, 44, 99
hypophosphataemia, 137
hypoproteinaemia, 143
hypospermia, 141
hypotension, 129, 132, 137, 144, 145
hypothyroidism, 44, 61, 85, 111, 134
hypotonia, 99
hypovitaminosis, 98, 159
hypoxia, 80

ibuprofen, 13, 33, 129, **130–1**
IL, 8, 15, 30, 47, 55, 59, 62, 69, 78, 93, 103, 113, 133, 139, 141, 142, 147
immunocompromise, 21, 144
immunodeficiency, 143
infection
  acute, 35, 36, 37, 60, 69, 71, 113, 120, 137, 140, 143, 144, 145, 146, 150, 153
  bacterial, 21, 35, 36, 37, 38, 47, 49, 82, 117, 120, 122
  chronic, 22, 35
  respiratory, 47, 49, 50, 51, 117
  viral, 50, 52, 76, 112, 117, 118
infliximab, 13, 28, 144
insomnia, 85, 113, 130, 137, 141
interleukin, *see* IL
interleukin inhibitors, *see* anti-IL
iron, 110, 111
ischaemia, 47, 50, 52, 58, 144

Jaccoud's arthropathy, 65, 66
Janus kinase, 13, 28, 33, 114, 139, 147
joint
  aspiration, 17, 21, 22, 23, 37, 41, 43, 45, 46, 70, **120**, 125
  cervical spine, 15, 31
  hip, 10, 14–19, 20–3, 31, 33, 44, 60, 61, 86, 89–92, 106, 125, 155, 159
  knee, 10, 14, 15–19, 20, 21, 26, 27, 31, 36, 38, 40, 44–6, 60, 70, 99, 102, 104, 106, 108, 152, 154, 155, 160

Kawasaki disease, 48, 52
keratoconjunctivitis, 74
keratoderma blennorrhagica, 36, 37
kyphosis, 89, 90, 95, 100, 155
  dorsal, 159
  thoracic, 31, 155

laxatives, 40, 132
laxity, 16, 65
leflunomide, 13, 28, 139, **143**
leucocytosis, 37, 53
leucopenia, 53, 64, 66, 129, 142, 145
LFTs, 11, 12, 22, 53, 67, 113, **114**, 139, 140, 141, 143, 146, 147
lissamine green test, 75, 76
livedo reticularis, 50, 67
liver function tests, *see* LFTs
Looser zone, 101
lumbar
  lordosis, 31, 155
  spine, 15, 31, 32, 94, 155, 159
  spondylosis, 32, 159
lymphoma, 10, 66, 75, 77, 118

macrocytic, 110, 111
macrophage, 8, 20, 25, 55, 62, 69, 78, 105, 107, 141, 144, 145
macrophage activation syndrome, *see* MAS
malaise, 21, 22, 36, 40, 50, 59, 60, 63, 72, 100
malar, 64, 65, 68
malignancy, 60, 61, 70, 72, 73, 77, 137, 142, 144, 146, 147, 150
MAS, 105, 107, 108
mastectomy, 110
meningitis, 65
meniscal injury, 15, 160
menorrhagia, 65
methicillin-resistant *Staphylococcus aureus*, *see* MRSA
methotrexate, 13, 28, 38, 46, 54, 58, 61, 68, 73, 82, 108, 111, 113, 114, 124, 133, 139, **140**, 144, 145, 147
microscopic polyangiitis, *see* MPA
migraine, 56, 63, 85, 145
miscarriage, 67
monophosphate dehydrogenase, 143
monozygotic, 103
MPA, 48, 49, 51, 52, 53, 118
MRSA, 22
myalgia, 51, 63, 65
myasthenia gravis, 141
mycophenolate mofetil (MMF), 68, 82, 83, 139, **143**
myeloma, 60, 61, 89, 90, 95, 101, 113
myeloperoxidase, 47, 118

myopathy, 119, 133, 142
drug-induced, 71, 72
inflammatory, 72
proximal, 99
myositis, 60, 71, 75

naloxone, 132
naproxen, 13, 33, 42, 129, **130–1**
nasolacrimal duct, 50
nasopharyngeal ulceration, 64
necrosis, 54, 66, 71, 133
neoplasm, 32, 118, 142, 147
nephritic syndrome, 51
nephrotic syndrome, 65
nephrotoxic, 114, 123, 140, 142, 143
neuralgia, 56
neutropenia, 129, 145, 146
neutrophils, 47, 59, 110, 112, 122, 133, 145, 147
non-opioid, 128
non-steroidal anti-inflammatory drug, *see* NSAID
NSAID, 12, 13, 19, 28, 33, 38, 42, 45, 46, 67, 76, 96, 106, 108, 111, 113, 128, **129–31**, 151

oedema, 24, 65, 70, 71, 79, 107, 125, 136, 137, 140, 141, 142, 145
oesophagus, 69, 135
oesophageal dysmotility, 70, 72, 79, 81
oesophagitis, 91, 135
oestrogen, 62, 67, 88, 136
onycholysis, 26, 105, 153, 156
opioid, 19, 87, 128, **131–2**
opsonin, 113
orthopaedic, 23, 120
osteoarthritis, *see* arthritis, osteo-
osteoblast, 8, 15, 88, 91, 92, 114, 135, 137, 138
osteoclast, 8, 15, 20, 25, 88, 91, 93, 135, 136, 137, 138, 141
osteomalacia, 61, 90, 95, **98–101**, 114, 115, 159
osteopenia, 8, 9, 66, 91, 101, 124, 136
osteoporosis, 8, 10, 16, 66, **88–92**, 95, 101, 107, 115, 125, 133, 134, **135–8**, 151, 152
osteosarcoma, 94
osteotomy, 96, 108
ototoxicity, 141
ovarian failure, premature, 92

Paget's disease, 16, 18, 90, **93–6**, 101, 114, 115, 135, 136, 137
PAN, **47–54**, 112, 134
pancytopenia, 66, 105
paraesthesia, 85, 99, 142, 145
paramyxovirus, 93
paraneoplastic, 81, 83
paraplegia, 94
paraprotein, 60
parathyroid
hormone (PTH), 90, 91, 98, 101, 115
peptide, 137
parotid, 74, 75, 76
penis, 36, 37
pericardial, 64, 66, 80, 83
pericarditis, 10, 64, 65, 105
periorbital, 70
phenytoin, 151
plantar, 71
fasciitis, 24, 27, 36
spurs, 37
PM, 61, **69–73**, 85, 117, 119, 133, 134
PMR, 55, 56, **59–61**, 85, 113, 126, 133, 134, 140, 142, 150
pneumonia, 70
pneumonitis, 124, 140, 142
podagra, 40
polyarteritis nodosa, *see* PAN
polyarthritis, 8, 9, 20, 40, 52, 75, 103, 120
polymyalgia rheumatica, *see* PMR
polymyositis, *see* PM
porphyria, 141, 142
post-menopausal, 16, 92, 136
PPI, 12, 19, 42, 61, 82, 89, 131, 134
pregabalin, 87, 128
pregnancy, 67, 99, 110, 123, 130, 132, 134, 135, 136, 137, 138, 140, 141, 142, 143, 144, 145, 146, 147
propylthiouracil, 47

prostaglandin, 129, 130
prostate, 101
prosthetic, 20, 21, 23, 120
proteinuria, 51, 64, 65, 66, 114, 143
proton pump inhibitors, *see* PPI
protozoa, 70
pseudogout, 15, 22, 41, 44, 150
  see also CPPD
psoriasis, 24–9, 31, 33, 104, 105, 141, 151
psychosis, 64, 140
punched-out erosions, 41
pyrexia, 50

quinolones, 47

radius, 88, 100
raloxifene, 92, 135, **136**
Raynaud's phenomenon, 65, 71, 75, 78, 79, 80, 81, 82
reactive arthritis, *see* arthritis, reactive
renal disease, 81, 82, 98, 119
rheumatoid arthritis, *see* arthritis, rheumatoid
rheumatologist, 12, 28
rhinorrhoea, 50
rickets, **98–102**, 114, 115
rifampicin, 98
Rinne's test, 95
rituximab, 13, 53, 68, 73, 76, 83, 139, **145**
romosozumab, 92, 135, **137–8**

sacroiliac (SI)
  joint, 24, 30, 32, 38
  pain, 31, 106
sacroiliitis, 24, 26, 27, 32, 36, 37
saddle nose, 50, 52, 54
Salmonella, 35
sarcoidosis, 75, 76, 92, 158
sciatica, 137, 159
scleritis, 10, 50, 51
sclerodactyly, 79, 82
scleroderma, 74, 75, **76–83**, 114, 116, 151
scleromyxoedema, 81
scoliosis, 155
secukinumab, 28, **146**
septic arthritis, *see* arthritis, septic
sequestosome, 93
sialography, 75, 76
sinusitis, 50, 51, 144
Sjögren's syndrome, 65, 70, **74–7**, 112, 117, 119, 150, 151
SLE, 11, 47, 49, **62–8**, 69, 72, 74, 75, 84, 111, 112, 113, 114, 116, 117, 118, 119, 122, 133, 134, 139, 141, 143, 150, 151, 152
smoking, 9, 11, 12, 42, 63, 64, 67, 88, 89, 91, 112, 152
spine pain, thoracic, 159
spondyloarthritis, 24, 30, 32, 35, 37, 38, 106, 113, 146, 147, 151, 158, 160
spondyloarthropathy, enteropathic, 24, 151
stiffness, 9, 16, 17, 26, 27, 31, 33, 34, 44, 59, 61, 80, 103, 104, 105, 108, 153, 159
  morning, 10, 11, 17, 18, 26, 33, 57, 59, 60, 65, 85, 106, 150
subluxation, atlanto-axial, 31
sulfasalazine, 13, 28, 38, 139, **141**, 151
swan neck deformity, 9, 156
syndesmophytes, 30, 32, 37
synovial, 8, 15, 20, 22, 59, 103, 145
  fluid, 15, 22, 23, 37, 39, 41, 44, 45, 46, 103, **120–2**
  hypertrophy, 8, 11, 15, 106, 107, 114
systemic lupus erythematosus, *see* SLE

tachycardia, 21, 22, 129, 145
tacrolimus, 67, 73
Takayasu's arteritis, 47–54
tenosynovitis, 60, 125, 143, 158
teratogen, 140, 143, 144
teriparatide, 91, 135, **137**, 138
thiazide, 40
thiopurine methyltransferase, *see* TPMT
thrombocytopenia, 53, 64, 66, 67, 68, 112, 129, 136, 142, 143
thrombocytosis, 37, 53, 56, 112, 147
thyroid, 60, 89, 90
T-lymphocyte, 35, 47, 62
TNF, 30, 103, 146
  alpha, 8, 13, 15, 28, 62, 69, 133, 141, 144, 146
  inhibitor, 13, 28, 33, 38, 108, 139, **144**, 147

tocilizumab, 13, 54, 58, 61, 108, 114, 139, **145**
TPMT, 142, 147
tramadol, 131, 132
tsDMARDs, 13, 139
tumour necrosis factor, *see* TNF
tyk2, 139

ulcer, 10, 21, 36, 37, 51, 52, 64, 65, 78, 80, 82, 111, 130, 133, 134, 135, 140, 142, 143, 145, 151
ulnar deviation, 9, 156, 157
ultrasound, 11, 22, 32, 41, 44, 45, 46, 53, 56, 57, 107, 120, 123, **124–5**
upadacitinib, 147
urticaria, 125, 145, 146
ustekinumab, 28
uveitis, 26, 31, 36, 51, 104, 106, 107, 119, 151

vaginal, 65, 74, 76
vancomycin, 22
vasculitis, **47–54**, 55, 68, 75, 112, 113, 114, 118, 126, 133, 140, 141, 142, 156
venepuncture, 110
vesiculobullous lesion, 52
vestibulocochlear nerve, 94
vitamin D deficiency, 58, 89, 90, 91, 96, **98–102**, 115

warfarin, 67
Weber's test, 95
Wegener's granulomatosis, *see* WG
WG, **47–54**, 116, 118, 145
Wilson's disease, 44

xerophthalmia, 74
xerostomia, 74
X-ray, 124

zoledronate, 91, 96, 135, 136
zoledronic acid, *see* zoledronate
Z-score, 90
Z-thumb, 9
zygapophyseal joint, 30